$\mathcal{A}$ROMATHERAPY

FOR HEALTH, WELL-BEING AND RELAXATION

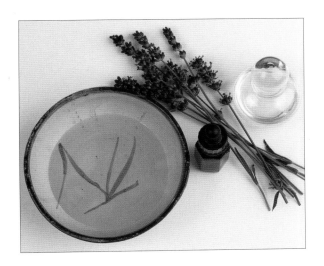

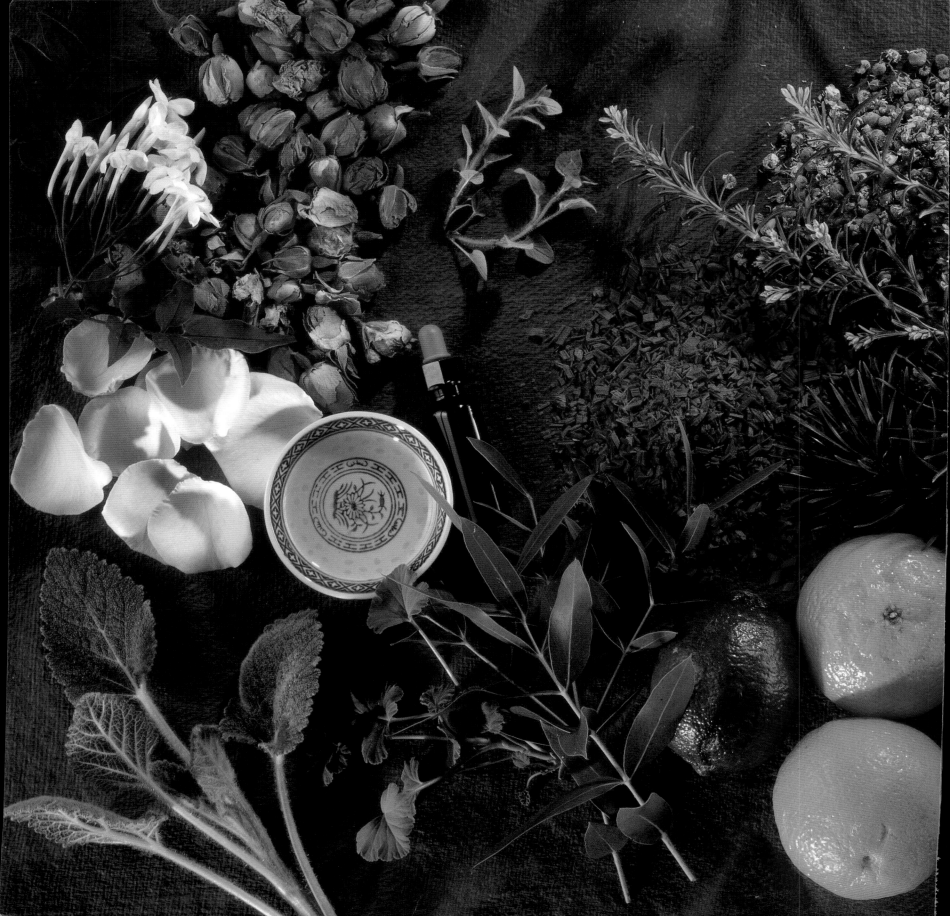

Aromatherapy

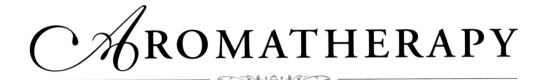

FOR HEALTH, WELL-BEING AND RELAXATION

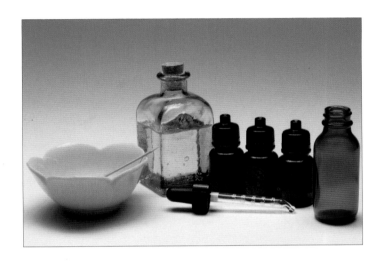

JOANNE RIPPIN

LORENZ BOOKS

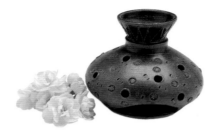

First published in the UK in 1997 by Lorenz Books

This edition published in the USA by Lorenz Books
27 West 20th Steet, New York, NY 10011; (800) 354-9657

LORENZ BOOKS are available for bulk purchase for sales promotion and for premium use.
For details write or call the sales director:
Lorenz Books, 27 West 20th Street, New York NY 10011; (800) 354-9657.

ISBN 1 85967 556 5

Publisher: Joanna Lorenz
Project Editor: Joanne Rippin
Editor: Beverley Jollands
Aromatherapy Consultant: Anita Glover
Designer: Lilian Lindblom

ACKNOWLEDGEMENTS
The publishers would especially like to thank Nitya Lacroix, Carole McGilvery, Jimi Reed and Sharon Seager who contributed the majority of the text in this book; also Andi Clevely, Mark Evans, Tessa Evelegh, Gilly Love, Alison Mackonochie, Sally Norton, Katherine Richmond, and Kate Shapland who supplied additional material.
The majority of photographs in the book were taken by Sue Atkinson and Alistair Hughes. Other photographs were taken by Simon Bottomley, Nick Cole, John Freeman, Michelle Garrett, Don Last and Debbie Patterson

Printed in Hong Kong / China

3 5 7 9 10 8 6 4 2

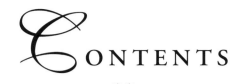CONTENTS

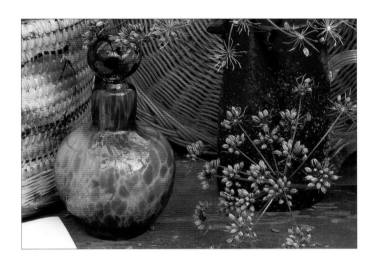

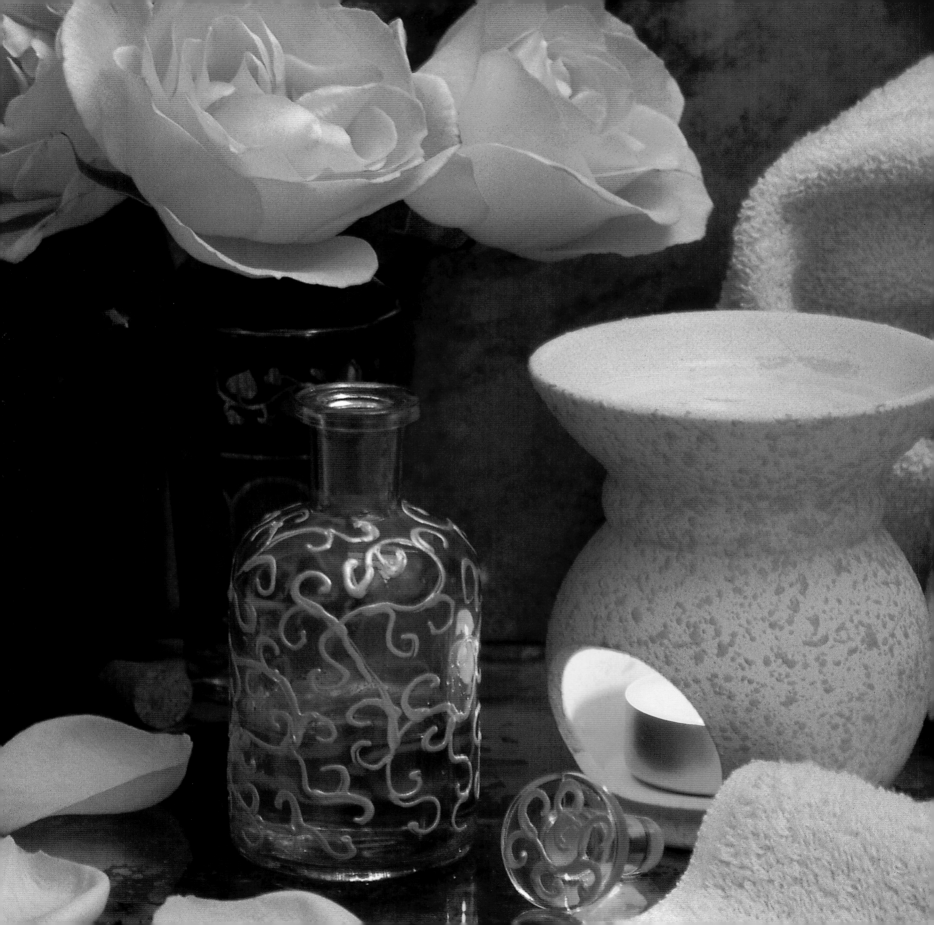

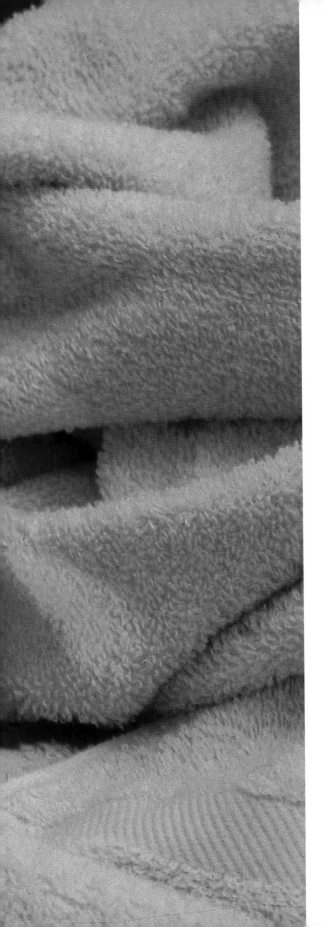

Introduction

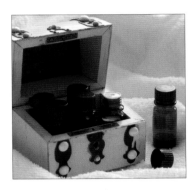

The value of natural plant oils has been recognized for more than 6000 years, because of their healing, cleansing, preservative and mood-enhancing properties, as well as the sheer pleasure of their fragrances. Today, these properties are being rediscovered as we look to the wisdom of past eras and civilizations to restore the balance that has been lost in modern life. Stress, pollution, unhealthy diet, hectic but sedentary lifestyles – all these factors have adverse effects on our bodies and spirits. The art of aromatherapy harnesses the pure essences of aromatic plants, flowers and resins, to work on the most powerful of the senses – smell and touch – to restore the harmony of body and mind. Use the beneficial properties of essential oils to treat common ailments, promote good health and emotional well-being, and to enhance every aspect of your life. These potent, volatile essences are nature's gift to mind and body.

THE HISTORY OF AROMATHERAPY

There is well-documented evidence from the great civilizations of the past to indicate that the use of herbs and aromatics in ancient times was commonplace, and that a large body of knowledge existed concerning the properties of these plants. During the intervening millennia much of this knowledge was lost or ignored, and it is only relatively recently that the wisdom of ancient healers in the application of essential oils has been rediscovered.

DISCOVERING THE SECRETS OF THE OILS

The origins of aromatherapy can be traced through the religious, medical and social practices of all the major civilizations. It is likely that the Chinese were the first to discover the remarkable medicinal powers of plants around 4500 BC. However, it is the Egyptians who must take the credit for recognizing and fully exploiting the physical and spiritual properties of aromatic essences.

From hieroglyphs and tomb paintings we know that aromatic preparations were used as offerings to the gods. Furthermore, the natural antiseptic and bactericidal properties of essential oils and resins, particularly cedarwood and frankincense, made them ideal for the purpose of preserving corpses in preparation for the next world. The discovery of remarkably well-preserved mummies up to 5000 years after their preparation is a tribute to the embalmer's art.

The Egyptians stored their raw materials in large clay or alabaster pots. Water was added and the pots heated so that steam rose and was pushed through a cotton cloth in the neck of the jar. This soaked up the essential oil which was then squeezed and pressed out into a collection vessel. The same principle remains in use in the sophisticated stills employed today.

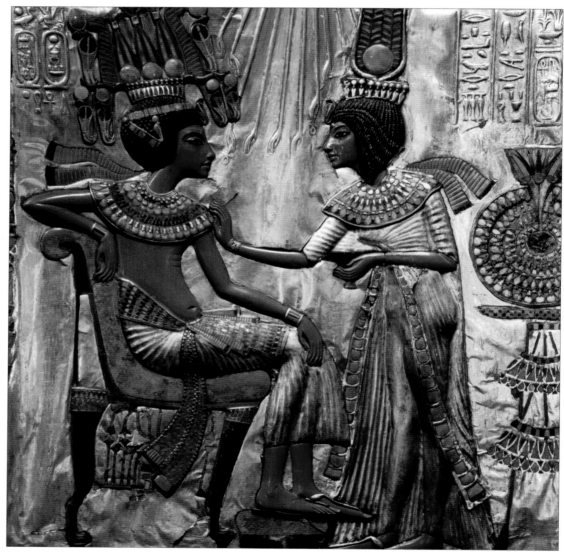

The back of Tutankhamun's throne shows the King being anointed with perfumed oil by his Queen, Ankhesenamun, 1357–1349 BC.

Aromatics in Therapy

By around 3000 BC Egyptian priests, who had been using the oils in religious ceremonies and embalming rites, became aware of the usefulness of their properties for the living. Closely guarding their secrets, they became the healers of their time, mixing and prescribing "magic" medicinal potions. The use of essential oils gradually permeated all levels of society as cosmetics and perfumes became widespread.

The Chinese, too, used aromatics for religious practices as well as for health, and applied them during massage as an additional means of maintaining a healthy body. The Chinese knowledge of herbs around 2500 BC is documented in *The Yellow Emperor's Classic of Internal Medicine*, traditionally said to have been written by the legendary Emperor Kiwang-Ti. More than 4000 years later in 1579, after 26 years of study, Le Shih-Chên published the Pên T'sao, an enormous and valuable volume in which he recorded the use of 2000 herbs and 20 essential oils. This book documents the greatest range of herbs studied in any tradition.

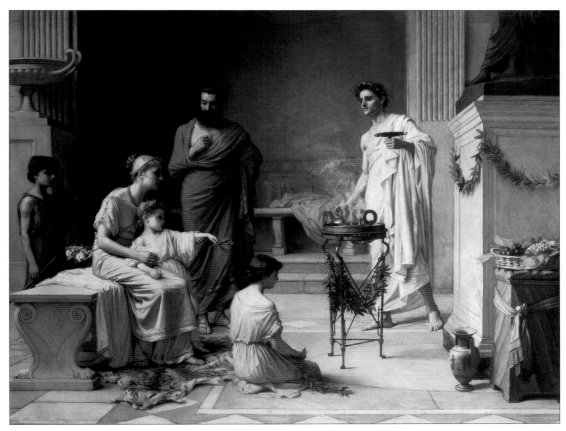

In ancient Greece the sick were treated with aromatic herbs and spices. Here fragrant herbs are burned in the temple of Asclepius to help a sick child.

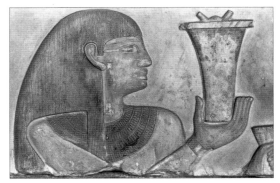

Many Egyptian paintings show perfume and ointment carriers being used in everyday life.

In India the traditional Ayervedic medical practice was developed from 2000-year-old texts, which list 700 useful aromatics, all valued for their spiritual and health-giving properties. There, as in China, the principal aspect of this form of medicine was the aromatic massage.

Aromatic substances were among the earliest traded goods, rare and highly prized. Phoenician merchants spread the trade of aromatic material into the Arabian peninsula and across the Mediterranean to Greece and Rome. The Greek physician Marestheus first recorded the stimulating and sedative qualities of different aromatic flowers, and in the first century AD Dioscorides compiled the *Herbarius*, a five-volume study of the sources and uses of plants and aromatics. This became the standard medical treatise for the following thousand years.

The Greeks and Romans used aromatics widely in rituals and ceremonies as well as in medicine, and the oils played an important role in the rise in popularity of baths, massage and body-culture generally throughout the Roman Empire. However, with the fall of the Empire in the fifth century the use of essential oils died out in Europe.

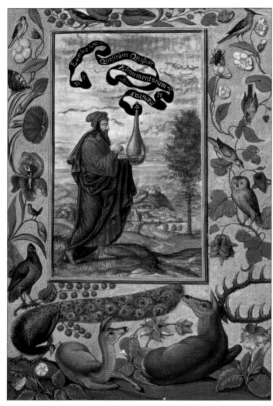

A sixteenth-century manuscript showing an alchemist. Much of the European herbalists' lore was adapted from the natural philosophy of the alchemists.

The development of perfumery

The art flourished elsewhere, though, particularly in Arabia, where Avicenna was the first to distil rose essence around AD 1000. Arabia became the world centre for the production of perfume, importing raw materials from Egypt, India, Tibet and China, and trading its products internationally.

The art of perfumery was reintroduced to Europe at the beginning of the twelfth century with the return of the first Crusaders. Records show that aromatics were used as protection against the plague and the low incidence of death among perfumers suggests they were to some degree effective. The fifteenth century saw the rise of the great European perfumers.

Revolutionary developments in science that began during the Renaissance led to the analysis and study of an increasing number of essential oils and other aromatic substances. A famous perfume industry developed in Grasse in the South of France, and by the end of the seventeenth century the distinction between apothecaries, who dealt with herbs for medicinal purposes, and the perfume manufacturers, had become quite pronounced.

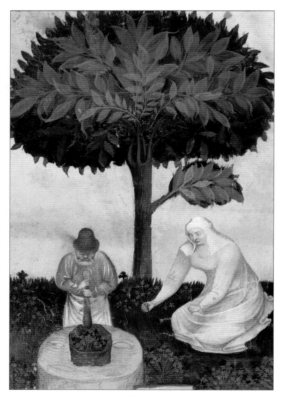

Fourteenth-century people had their own herbal lore, and were skilled at gathering and processing certain plants for medical or culinary purposes.

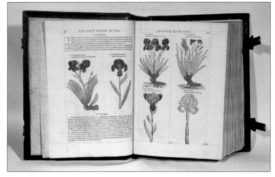

One of the first books on herbalism by John Gerard: these pages show the flower-de-luce.

Herbalism

The advent of mechanized printing allowed the publication of popular herbals making texts such as Banckes' *Herbal* (1527) available to a wider public. In seventeenth-century England, Nicholas Culpeper, John Parkinson and John Gerard, among others, led the way in the golden age of English herbalism. At the same time, natural philosophy that had been such an important part of the alchemists' work was left behind, to be developed in isolation by artists and thinkers. This development marked the beginning of the separation of body and spirit that is so evident in medical practice today.

During this time, as scientific knowledge about essential oils grew, their use in medicine became less important, and the concept of holism was lost, albeit temporarily. In the mid-seventeenth century the separation between traditional herbalists and physicians who favoured chemical drug therapy began. However, philosophers exploring alchemy further refined the art of distillation, allowing more and more aromatic essences to be created for a wide range of uses.

THE MODERN ART AND PRACTICE OF AROMATHERAPY

The French doctor and scientist René-Maurice Gattefossé is the twentieth-century father of aromatherapy. Gattefossé is credited with coining the name "aromatherapy" to describe treatments with essential oils. His interest was aroused as the result of an accident he sustained while working in the laboratory of a perfumery. He burnt his hand badly and plunged it into the nearest available liquid, which happened to be essential oil of lavender. The burns healed very quickly with minimal scarring, prompting him to research into the healing qualities of this and other essential oils. He also discovered that essential oils are more powerful in their natural state than when their active chemicals are used in isolation. Gattefossé published the results of his findings in his book *Aromathérapie* (1937).

Many of those who came after Gattefossé helped to rediscover the link between the mind and spirit and a healthy body. The Frenchman Jean Valnet, also a doctor and scientist, used essential oils to treat wounds during the Second World War, as well as to treat specific illnesses. Today in France there are many medical doctors prescribing essential oils for internal use to heal ailments.

Valnet's work was taken up and developed by Madame Marguerite Maury, a beauty therapist who was interested in incorporating essential oils into her treatments. Her principle was to revitalize each client by using a personal aromatic blend, which she based on the individual's temperament and specific health disorders.

Madame Maury was dissatisfied with the

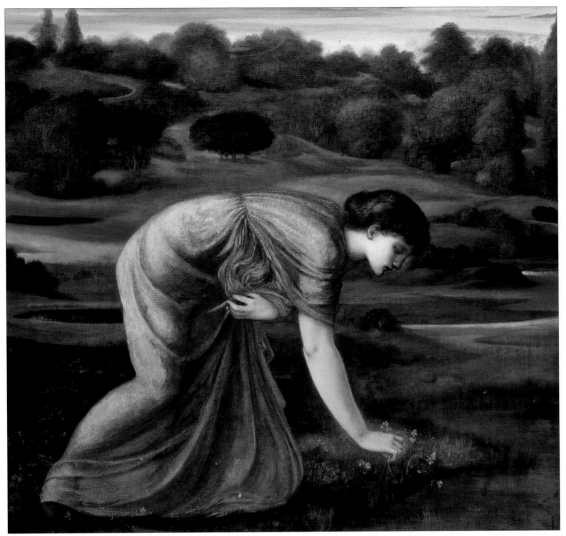

Practitioners of the healing arts relied on plants to heal illness for thousands of years. Many of the herbs they commonly used are plants from which essential oils are extracted.

oral administration of essential oils, and rediscovered the method of applying them in diluted form during massage, as had been practised by the ancient healers.

Today, widespread use is made of aromatherapy in many fields of conventional medicine. Aromatherapy has been found to be useful in alleviating the symptoms for patients suffering long-term illnesses such as cancer and AIDS. Most imaginatively, it has recently been used by volunteers working with orphaned children in Romania, and one enterprising South African teacher uses essential oils to create a calm atmosphere of learning and concentration in her township nursery school.

THE ESSENTIAL OILS

An essential oil is the essence or personality of a plant, the plant's life force distilled for use. The fragrance and character of each oil are as individual and unique as a fingerprint, as are its therapeutic properties and the effects they have on the individual. Essential oils are natural, volatile substances that evaporate readily, quickly releasing their aroma into the air, as happens, for example, when someone brushes against an aromatic plant in a garden. The German term for essential oils means "ethereal oils", which is a much more accurate and evocative description. Some 300 essential oils are commercially available, but of these only between 50 and 100 have health-giving properties and are suitable for use in aromatherapy.

SOURCES OF ESSENTIAL OILS

Not all plants contain essential oils. In those that do, the oil, or essence, is contained in highly specialized glands that are present in the foliage, flower or other part of the plant. The purpose of the oil is to help prevent water loss from the plant. As the oils evaporate they create a barrier around the leaf or other part and so reduce evaporation. Essential oils may also provide some defence against infection, and attract insects that are vital to pollination.

The plants that contain essential oils are found mainly in hot, dry habitats. In some plants, such as marjoram, the essential oil glands are present in the minute hairs on the leaves, but in woody plants such as rosewood they are embedded in the fibrous bark or wood. In others the oil glands can be seen clearly as shiny, coloured disks on the surface of the leaf or flower.

At certain times of the day, and particular times of the year, the essential oils are present at optimum levels, and this is the best time for harvest and distillation. The amount of oil produced by a plant is also affected by the growing conditions, including the type of soil, the amount of sunlight it receives, and

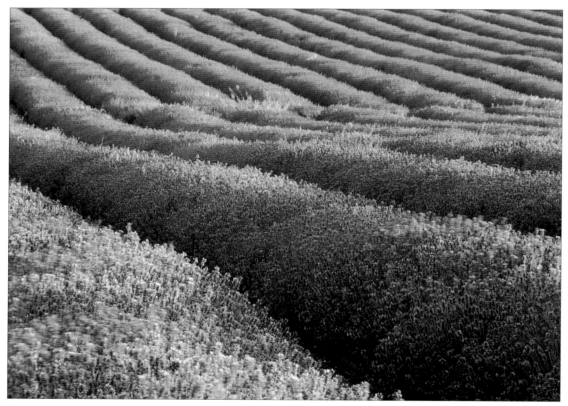

French lavender produces a fruitier, sweeter aroma than English lavender, which has a camphorous undertone. It takes 1 tonne/1 ton of plants to yield about 9 kg/20 lb of essential oil.

rainfall. French lavender, for example, is famous for its rich aroma but, like wine, the quality can vary from year to year.

Essential oils have a consistency similar to that of water and most are lighter than water,

although some are heavier. All of them differ from vegetable oils in that they are not greasy. Most are colourless; those that are coloured include bergamot, which is green, lemon oil, which is yellow, and chamomile, blue.

CHEMICAL CONSTITUENTS

A particular oil may contain between 50–500 different chemicals. Rose oil contains the greatest number, some of which are found in such minute quantities that they have not yet been identified. This has made it impossible to reproduce accurately the most exquisite of all essential oils.

Each of the many chemicals present in an essential oil has its own properties, which are in turn imparted to the oil. The chemical complexity of essential oils is responsible for their various characteristics and the actions they produce in the body.

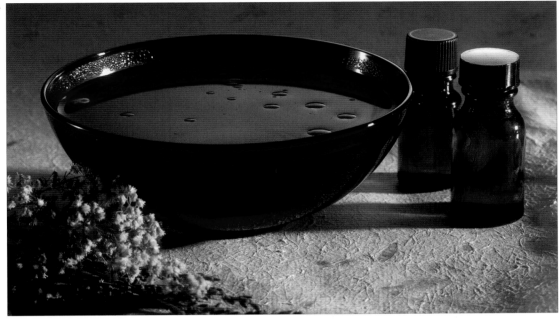

Essential oils evaporate readily: a few drops added to hot water will fragrance a room.

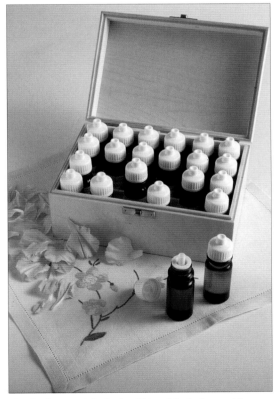

Bottles for essential oils should be of dark glass and have a stopper incorporating a drop dispenser. Keep the bottles tightly closed, and away from direct light and heat.

HOW ESSENTIAL OILS WORK

Essential oils are composed of tiny molecules which are easily dissolved in alcohol, emulsifiers and, particularly, fats. This allows them to penetrate the skin easily and work into the body by mixing with the fatty tissue.

As these highly volatile essences evaporate they are also inhaled, thus entering the body via the millions of sensitive cells that line the nasal passages. These send messages straight to the brain, and affect the emotions by working on the limbic system, which also controls the major functions of the body.

The chemicals in essential oils unleash the body's ability to heal. They are carried to all parts in the blood, after which they are excreted through the lungs and in the urine. Diluting the oils delays their passage through the body but does not detract from their efficacy. After a treatment, the essential oil remains in the body for 3–4 hours, activating the healing process, which can continue for 2–3 weeks.

Essential oils are able to influence all aspects of the body's functions, from tissues to organs, to body fluids and cells, as well as the emotional state and the spiritual aspects of the person.

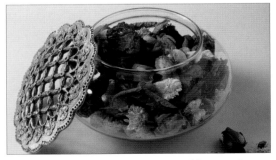

Essential oils are used to scent a variety of fragrant objects, such as candles, potpourri and pomanders.

EXTRACTING ESSENTIAL OILS

Most essential oils are produced by distillation or expression. Generally, because of the fragile nature of the raw material, the processing takes place in the country of origin. More robust materials, such as wood, bark, and seeds, are sometimes exported for distillation elsewhere. Herbs and flowers can be distilled fresh or dried, and hardier material such as wood needs to be chipped or even powdered before processing can begin. The citrus oils, contained in the peel of the fruit, are all expressed (squeezed), often by hand. Other essential oils are produced by dry, water or steam distillation.

Distillation

The commonest method of production is steam distillation. By this method the volatile and water-soluble parts are separated from the rest of the plant. The resulting mixture may need to be distilled a second time to remove non-volatile matter.

In the distillation process the plant is placed in a sealed container. Water in a second container is heated to produce steam, which is passed under pressure through the plant material. The steam causes the glands containing the essence to burst, allowing the volatile chemicals to dissolve in the steam. This rises and is taken into a condensing chamber, where it is cooled. As it cools and condenses the essential oil is separated from the water. Floral water is a by-product of distilling and, like essential oil, has therapeutic and commercial uses.

Solvent Extraction

A lengthier and more expensive process, solvent extraction is favoured for releasing essential oil from more delicate material, such as jasmine flowers. The plant material is washed with a solvent such as alcohol until the essence dissolves. The resulting material is then distilled at a precise, quite low, temperature to separate the solvent and the aromatic oil. Oil made by this process is known as an absolute.

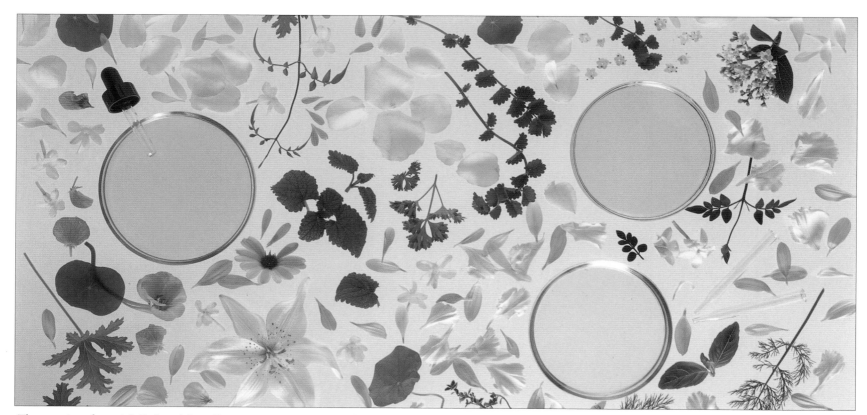

The extraction of essential oils from delicate flowers is a time-consuming and costly process.

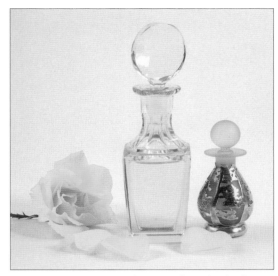

Store blends of essential and carrier oils in glass bottles, securely stoppered.

BUYING THE FINEST OILS

For the best results use only the finest oils. In general, price is an excellent guide to quality, and it is wise to compare various suppliers' prices so that you can recognize an extremely expensive oil and an unbelievably cheap one. Be aware that essential oils are easily adulterated, and do not be misled by unscrupulous marketing practices. For example, there is no such thing as cheap rose oil; cheap rose oil is probably a similar-smelling product to which geranium or palmarosa oil has been added. Rosemary may also be adulterated, by the addition of camphor or eucalyptus.

If you buy from a reputable source you will also avoid those unscrupulous manufacturers who, although offering a pure essential oil, market oils from a second or third distillation. These will contain only a few active ingredients; the majority will have been removed during the first processing.

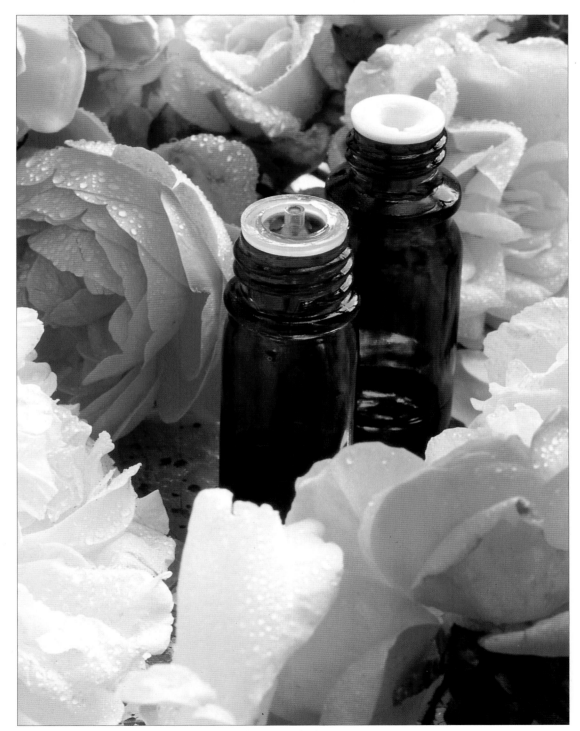

Rose is one of the most expensive and complex of all the essential oils.

THE MECHANICS OF SMELLING

When a scent is inhaled, the odour molecules float to the back of the nasal cavity, where they dissolve and unite with receptor, or olfactory, cells. These trigger off electrical signals via the nerve pathways to the olfactory bulb in the brain. Only eight molecules of scent are needed to trigger the smell mechanism. Most of the essential oil molecules that have triggered the system are breathed out, although some will enter the bloodstream via the lungs and will then travel around the body for several hours before they are eliminated.

The areas of the brain to which messages concerning smell are sent are the cerebral cortex and the limbic system. The limbic system controls many vital activities such as sleep, sexual drive, hunger and thirst as well as smell. This is also the area of the brain that

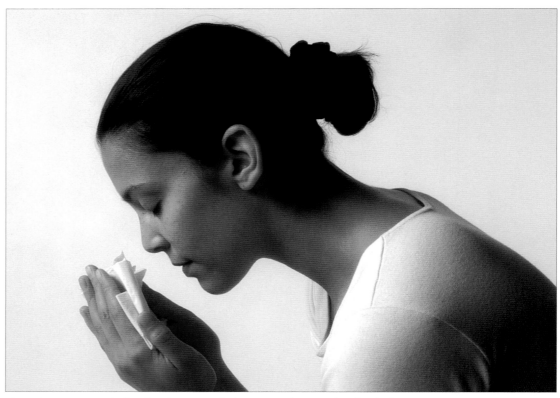

A simple way to enjoy the benefits of an essential oil is to put a drop on a handkerchief.

relates to emotion and memory, which gives the clue to the link between smell, emotion and memory. Odours also connect with the hypothalamus, which controls the endocrine system and nervous system. Through this mechanism the brain comes into contact with the outside world. Specific neuro-chemicals within the nervous system are stimulated by the different scents.

The apparent fading of a scent occurs when all the receptor cells are full, but after ten minutes or so they are vacated and can be reoccupied, causing the scent to "come back". This explains why we fail to notice a scent if we have been exposed to it for a while, while it may smell strong to someone just coming into the room.

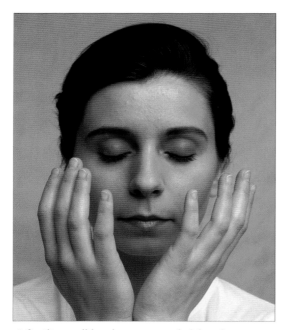

A familiar smell has the power to unlock long-lost memories.

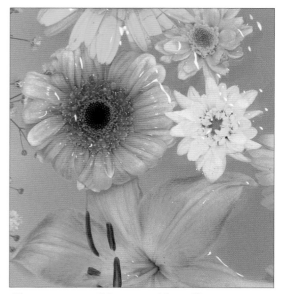

Pleasant aromas will have an uplifting effect on your emotional state.

CAUTIONS: Essential oils are highly concentrated substances and must be used with caution. Follow the points listed below and for the treatment of persistent problems, ask the advice of a qualified aromatherapist. If in any doubt, seek a medical opinion before using essential oils.

• Never take essential oils internally, unless professionally prescribed.

• Always use essential oils diluted. Do not exceed the recommended rates: up to 3-6 drops essential oil to 10 ml/2 tsp carrier oil; just 5 drops in a bath or for a steam inhalation.

• Do not use the same oils for more than one or two weeks at any one time.

• When mixing your own blends, do not use more than three oils in any one treatment as the synergistic effects are less predictable.

• Do not use oils in pregnancy without getting professional advice. The following oils are contra-indicated at this time: bay, basil, clary sage, comfrey, fennel, hyssop, juniper, marjoram, melissa, myrrh, rosemary, sage and thyme.

• For anyone with skin problems, dilute the oils even more and, if any skin irritation occurs, stop using them immediately. A few essential oils, such as bergamot, make the skin more sensitive to sunlight, so should be used with caution in hot, sunny weather.

• Be extra careful with anyone who has asthma or epilepsy and if they experience a reaction, stop using the oil.

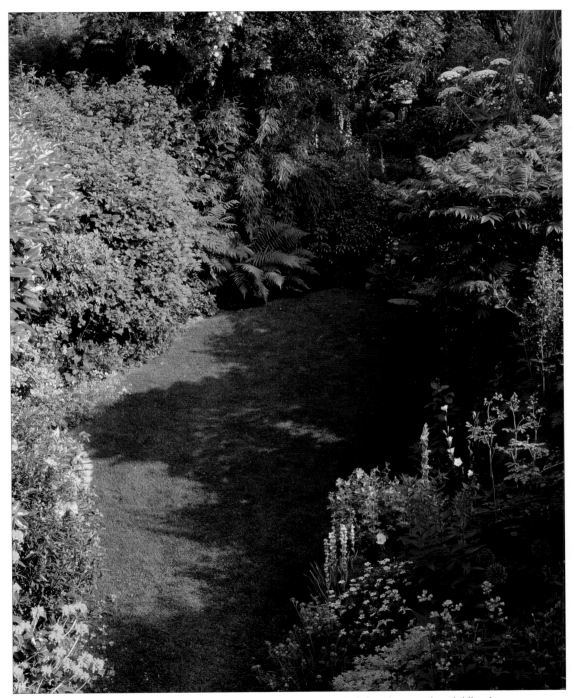

A fragrance may conjure up a vivid image from the past – perhaps of a secluded garden visited in childhood. Both memory and emotion are linked to our sense of smell; all three are governed by the same area of the brain, the limbic system.

CHOOSING THE RIGHT OILS

The essential oils profiled in the following pages play a major part in the aromatherapist's practice and constitute the principal oils suitable for use in the home. Use the detailed descriptions of their effects to help you choose an oil or put together a blend that will suit your particular needs.

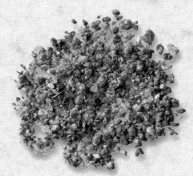

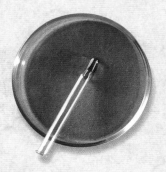

BENZOIN
Styrax benzoin

Benzoin is a warming and comforting oil produced from the sap of a tall tree native to tropical Asia. It is one of the ingredients in Friar's Balsam, a mixture used to treat respiratory complaints. It was also, together with lavender and ethanol, one of the main ingredients in an old-fashioned toilet water called Virgin's Milk, which reputedly left the skin "clear and brilliant". Like sandalwood, it is a traditional ingredient in incense.

APPLICATIONS AND EFFECTS

Calming and soothing. Particularly effective for respiratory conditions and mental and emotional disorders.

Skin: Cracked, dry and chapped skin, also wrinkled skin, chilblains, rashes, wounds, sores, itching; soothing to irritation resulting from sunburn, rashes and hives.

Circulatory and muscular systems: Arthritis, gout, poor circulation, muscular aches and pains, rheumatism.

Respiratory system: Bronchitis (very effective on congested mucous membranes), chills, chesty coughs, sore throats and laryngitis.

Digestive system: Flatulence, colic.

Immune system: 'Flu, cystitis, mouth ulcers.

Nervous system: Insomnia, nervous tension, bed-wetting.

Mental/emotional effects: Calms stress and tension, comforts sad, lonely and depressed individuals. Helps to let go of worries, gives confidence and helps in exhausted emotional and psychic states.

CAUTION: Can cause drowsiness.

BERGAMOT
Citrus bergamia

Bergamot is an ornamental citrus tree native to tropical Asia. The peel of the ripe fruit yields an oil that is mild and gentle, with a sweet, aromatic odour. It is one of the main constituents of eau-de-Cologne and lavender water, and is also found in some sun-tan preparations. The plant is now cultivated in Italy and on the Ivory Coast and its common name may have come from the city of Bergamo in northern Italy. Bergamot leaves are used to flavour Earl Grey tea. Not to be confused with the herb bergamot (*Monarda didyma*).

APPLICATIONS AND EFFECTS

Particularly effective for boils, eczema, psoriasis, anxiety and depression.

Skin: Acne, cold sores, insect bites, insect repellent, oily complexions (especially stress-related), spots, wounds.

Respiratory system: Bad breath, sore throat, tonsillitis, bronchitis.

Digestive system: Flatulence, poor appetite (has a regulating action, which may be useful for anorexia), colic, indigestion.

Reproductive and excretory systems: Cystitis, thrush.

Nervous system: PMS (mood swings), insomnia, nightmares.

Immune system: Colds, 'flu, fever, cold sores, chicken pox, immune deficiency, herpes.

Mental/emotional effects: Its cooling and refreshing action helps soothe anger and frustration. Bergamot is useful for grief; the uplifting nature of this oil makes the bereaved receptive to joy and love again.

CAUTION: Not to be used before going out into the sun, even when diluted, as it can cause discoloration of the skin that results in a rash.

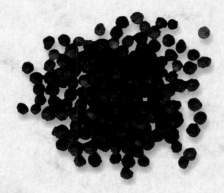

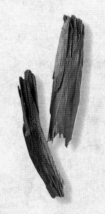

BLACK PEPPER
Piper nigrum

The essential oil of black pepper comes from the fruit of a tropical vine. These fruits are the same peppercorns used for culinary purposes, the familiar spice commonly added to food. The vine, which has heart-shaped leaves and white blooms, is extensively cultivated in South-east Asia. Black pepper is one of the three oldest-known spices, the other two being cloves and cinnamon. The oil is warming and comforting and surprisingly sweet; it can often add a mysterious depth to a blend. In ancient times it was very highly valued: it is said of Attila the Hun that he demanded black pepper as part of the ransom for Rome.

APPLICATIONS AND EFFECTS

Particularly effective for muscular aches and pains, fevers, colds, 'flu.
Skin: Chilblains.
Circulatory and muscular systems: Arthritis, neuralgia, poor circulation, rheumatic pain, sprains, stiffness, poor muscle tone.
Respiratory system: Catarrh, chills. Used as a homeopathic remedy, it can relieve fevers.
Digestive system: Colic, constipation, sluggish digestion, diarrhoea, flatulence, heartburn, loss of appetite, nausea.
Immune system: Colds, 'flu, infections caused by bacteria (urinary, respiratory or digestive), viral infections.
Mental/emotional effects: Gives stamina where there is frustration, and enthusiasm where there is indifference. Can help where there is lack of interest and vitality, such as when recovering from an infection.

CAUTION: Care should be taken by those with sensitive skins, as in high concentrations it can occasionally cause irritation. Too frequent use may over-stimulate the kidneys.

CEDARWOOD
Cedrus atlantica

Cedar is a Semitic word meaning "the power of spiritual strength". The tree from which the essential oil is extracted is native to the Atlas mountains of Morocco, but it is now grown more widely, particularly in Lebanon and some parts of the Far East. The majestically tall, pyramid-shaped evergreen gives an oil that embodies the ancient qualities of its name – confidence and firmly rooted spiritual strength. The oil is extracted by steam distillation from the wood of the tree. It was used in ancient times by the Egyptians in the form of a gum, as a main ingredient for the preservation of mummies, and it is thought to be one of the earliest-known oils. The oil is still used by Tibetans as a temple incense and by natives of North Africa for medicinal purposes.

APPLICATIONS AND EFFECTS

Particularly effective for long-standing complaints rather than acute ones; has aphrodisiac properties.
Skin: Acne, dandruff.
Circulatory and muscular systems: Arthritis, rheumatism, poor circulation.
Respiratory system: Bronchitis, catarrh, coughs, chest infections.
Reproductive and excretory systems: Cystitis.
Mental/emotional effects: This uplifting oil is useful for lack of confidence or fearfulness. It has euphoric properties that help to eliminate mental stagnation in depressed states. It is relaxing and soothing and can be a good aid to meditation.

CAUTION: Best avoided during pregnancy.

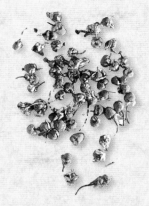

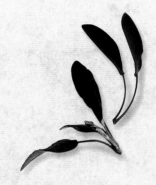

CHAMOMILE
Anthemis nobilis

There is a long tradition of use for this gentle yet strengthening herb. The Moors and Egyptians recognized its calming qualities and the Saxons used it as part of their mixture of nine sacred herbs in an incense known as "maythen". There are several varieties of chamomile from which essential oils are obtained, but the most commonly used are Roman chamomile (*Anthemis nobilis*) and German chamomile (*Matricaria chamomilla*). They have similar properties, although they differ in appearance. Roman chamomile is a creeping perennial with tiny, needle-like leaves; German chamomile is a taller, upright annual with fragile, feathery leaves. Both have small, white, daisy-like flowers. The essential oil of German chamomile has a larger proportion of the anti-inflammatory chemical azulene, which is useful for treating skin conditions.

APPLICATIONS AND EFFECTS
Calming. Particularly effective for teething pain, headaches.
Skin: Acne, allergies, boils, burns, chilblains, earache, inflammations, insect bites, toothache.
Circulatory and muscular systems: Arthritis, muscular pain, rheumatism, sprains.
Digestive system: Colic, indigestion, nausea.
Reproductive and excretory systems: Painful periods, menopause, PMS, cystitis.
Immune system: Thrush, fever.
Nervous system: Insomnia, nervous tension, bed-wetting.
Mental/emotional effects: A gently sedative oil for the highly strung and over-enthusiastic. Useful where symptoms are related to anger, irritability or unexpressed emotions.

CAUTION: Some people may find it causes dermatitis.

CLARY SAGE
Salvia sclarea

This tall, biennial herb grows in most parts of the world and provides a powerful aromatic, yet benevolent, euphoric oil. Its leaves are rather similar to those of common sage, although they are broader, wrinkled and hairy. The blue-white flowers are smaller than those of the more familiar herb and are enclosed in greeny-yellow, sometimes purplish, bracts. The Latin name *salvia* means "good health" and *sclarea* means "clear". Because of its euphoric properties it was sometimes substituted for hops in the brewing of beer. Today it is more widely used as a culinary herb in soups and stews as well as in the perfume industry.

APPLICATIONS AND EFFECTS
Particularly effective for reproductive and excretory disorders.
Skin: Acne, boils, dandruff.
Circulatory and muscular systems: High blood pressure, muscular aches and pains.
Respiratory system: Throat infections.
Digestive system: Colic, cramp, flatulence.
Reproductive and excretory systems: Irregular or painful periods, PMS, menopausal problems.
Immune system: Myalgic encephalomyelitis (ME), convalescence.
Nervous system: Depression, migraine, nervous tension, insomnia, panic.
Mental/emotional effects: Useful for difficulty in adjusting to change. Helps put things into perspective. Encourages dream recall; may help the individual to see more clearly.

CAUTION: Should be avoided by pre-menopausal women with a history of breast, cervical, ovarian or uterine cancer. May cause problems in some women taking the contraceptive pill or hormone replacement therapy (HRT). Avoid using with alcohol as it may exaggerate the effects or cause nausea. Not to be used before driving.

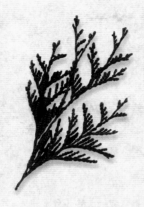

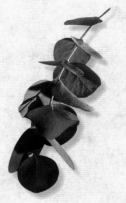

CYPRESS
Cupressus sempervirens

EUCALYPTUS
Eucalyptus globulus

The cypress tree is a statuesque evergreen that grows wild in southern France, Italy, Spain, Portugal, Corsica and North Africa. The specific Latin name *sempervirens* means "everlasting", and both the Egyptians and Romans dedicated it to their deities of the underworld. The essential oil is yellow and has a rich scent similar to the scent of pine needles. It is extracted from the cones of the plant by steam distillation; the main centres of production are in Europe, in Germany and France.

Some 15 species of this tall evergreen tree yield a useful essential oil. They include *Eucalyptus citriadoria* and *E. radiata*, as well as *E. globulus*. The leaves and oil of the plant have long been a household remedy in Australia, where the aborigines, who know it as "kino", use it to dress wounds. The young trees, which have round, bluish leaves, are valued by florists and gardeners. As the plants mature the foliage becomes long, narrow and yellowish in colour. The flowers are white and the smooth bark is often covered with a white bloom.

APPLICATIONS AND EFFECTS

Useful when there is an excess of fluids in some way. Particularly effective for diarrhoea, water retention and runny colds.

Skin: Oily and puffy skin, sweaty feet (when blended with peppermint), wounds.

Circulatory and muscular systems: Cellulite, muscular cramps, poor circulation, rheumatism.

Respiratory system: Bronchitis, spasmodic coughing, 'flu.

Digestive system: Haemorrhoids.

Reproductive and excretory systems: Heavy and painful periods, menopausal problems, cystitis.

Nervous system: Nervous tension.

Mental/emotional effects: The solemn nature of cypress makes it useful during periods of transition such as bereavement. It is also helpful at times for feelings of sadness and self-pity. It can be useful for soothing anger and quietening over-talkative people. It is spiritually cleansing and aids the removal of psychic blocks.

CAUTION: Should be used with caution during pregnancy.

APPLICATIONS AND EFFECTS

Useful in congested and toxic states. Particularly effective for muscular aches, bronchitis, colds, coughs, sinusitis and throat infections.

Skin: Insect bites, insect repellent.

Circulatory and muscular systems: Poor circulation, arthritis.

Reproductive and excretory systems: Cystitis, diarrhoea.

Nervous system: Headaches.

Immune system: 'Flu, fevers.

Mental/emotional effects: This oil has a deeply grounding quality, which can help cool overheated emotions. Its cleansing and harmonizing nature makes it useful where there has been emotional or physical conflict, and for places that just feel uncomfortable. It may also aid concentration.

CAUTION: Some people may find it irritates the skin.

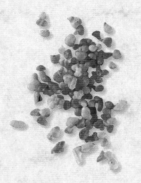
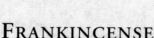
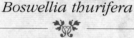

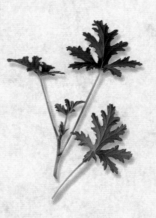

FRANKINCENSE
Boswellia thurifera

Frankincense (also known as olibanum) is an inspiring and contemplative oil that comes from the gum of a small tree or shrub grown mainly in the Middle East, with most of the oil produced in Iran and Lebanon. The gum is extracted by incising the trunk and peeling away the bark. The oozing juice slowly hardens on contact with the air and is then collected for distillation. The gum was highly prized in ancient times and was known simply by the old French name *franc encens*, "frank" meaning high quality. Frankincense is familiar primarily from its biblical connection as one of the three gifts to the infant Jesus: at that time its value was almost as great as that of gold. In ancient Egypt it was used as an incense in religious ceremonies and in cosmetics, where it was valued for its rejuvenating properties.

APPLICATIONS AND EFFECTS
Particularly effective for mature skin, bronchitis and anxiety.
Skin: Dry skin, scars, wounds, sores, ulcers.
Respiratory system: Catarrh, coughs, laryngitis, rheumatic conditions.
Reproductive and excretory systems: Cystitis, painful periods, heavy periods.
Immune system: Colds, 'flu.
Nervous system: Nervous tension, fear, nightmares.
Mental/emotional effects: Regulating oil, yet stimulating. This makes it useful in cases of exhaustion and mental fatigue. Useful for those who lack confidence and are weary of spirit. An excellent aid to meditation, as it deepens and slows the breath.

GERANIUM
Pelargonium graveolens

This adaptable oil has been widely used since antiquity, when it was thought to keep evil spirits at bay. The essential oil is strong when pure but sweetens when diluted. It comes from a perennial shrub covered in tiny hairs, which bears small pink flowers and has pointed, serrated leaves from which the essential oil is obtained, though all parts of the plant are scented. The plant is native to Africa, but is now cultivated in many parts of the world, as a house plant as well as commercially for its oil. Production of the oil is centred mainly in Réunion; other producers include France, Italy, China and Egypt.

APPLICATIONS AND EFFECTS
Particularly effective for sluggish, oily complexions and combination skin, irregular menstrual periods, mood swings and post-natal depression.
Skin: Acne, bruises, burns, chilblains, dermatitis, eczema, herpes, wounds.
Circulatory and muscular systems: Cellulite, poor circulation, fluid retention, detoxifying the body.
Respiratory system: Sore throats, tonsillitis.
Reproductive and excretory systems: PMS, menopause, urinary infections.
Nervous system: Nervous tension, diarrhoea resulting from a nervous condition, anxiety, depression.
Mental/emotional effects: Balancing, harmonizing and cleansing. Can be stimulating and uplifting. A useful alternative to bergamot as an anti-depressant oil.

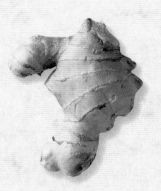

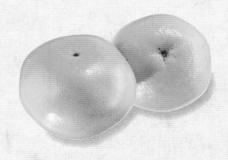

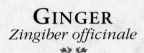

GINGER
Zingiber officinale

Like benzoin, the essential oil of ginger is known for its warm, comforting nature. The oil is extracted from the dried tuberous root of a plant that is native to south Asia. The plant itself has a reed-like stalk with narrow, spear-shaped leaves and yellow or white flowers that are carried on a spike rising straight from the tuber. There is some debate as to the derivation of its name. The Greeks called it *ziggiber*, and in Sanskrit writings it is listed as *srngavera*. However, its name may come from the area called Gingi, where it was drunk as a tea to cure stomachache.

APPLICATIONS AND EFFECTS

Quintessentially balancing; counteracts ailments caused by dampness. Particularly effective for muscular aches and pains, catarrh, coughs and colds (especially runny colds).
Skin: Clears bruises.
Circulatory and muscular systems: Poor circulation, rheumatism, sprains, strains.
Respiratory system: Congestion, sinusitis, chills.
Digestive system: Diarrhoea, colic, cramp, flatulence, indigestion, hangovers, loss of appetite, nausea, travel sickness.
Reproductive and excretory systems: Regulates menstruation after colds.
Immune system: Fever, 'flu, infectious disease, sore throat.
Nervous system: Debility, nervous exhaustion or fatigue.
Mental/emotional effects: This oil is comforting and grounding at the same time. When emotions are flat and cold it can be used to warm them. Ginger sharpens the senses and memory.

CAUTION: May be slightly phototoxic. In high concentrations it may cause skin irritation.

GRAPEFRUIT
Citrus paradisi

The grapefruit tree is cultivated for its delicious, large, yellow fruits. The tree reaches about 10 m/33 ft in height, and bears dark, glossy leaves and white flowers. It is native to tropical Asia and the West Indies, although it probably originated in Asia as a hybrid of the orange tree. Grapefruit trees are grown as ornamental trees all over the Mediterranean and are also cultivated in Florida, Brazil and Israel. California is the main producer of the oil. The yield of oil from the fresh peel is small when compared to the yields from the orange and lemon. Like other citrus oils it has a relatively short shelf life.

APPLICATIONS AND EFFECTS

Cleansing, balancing, brightening and refreshing. Particularly effective for congested pores and oily skin, cellulite, and the digestion of fatty foods.
Skin: Acne.
Circulatory and muscular systems: Muscle fatigue, exercise preparation, stiffness, water retention, migraine.
Digestive system: Loss of appetite, cleansing the kidneys, liver tonic.
Reproductive and excretory systems: PMS.
Immune system: Chills, colds, flu.
Nervous system: Depression, headaches, migraine, performance stress, nervous exhaustion, jet lag, restoration of balance after ear infections.
Mental/emotional effects: Use this uplifting oil when feeling apathetic or indecisive. Its euphoric nature may help with feelings of resentfulness, jealousy and envy.

CAUTION: Presents a very slight risk of producing photosensitivity in the skin.

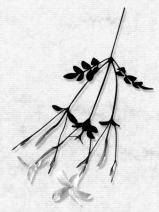

JASMINE
Jasminum officinale

Described as "the king of flower oils" and "the scent of angels", jasmine is renowned as an aphrodisiac and is often used in love potions. It is a tall evergreen vine with bright green leaves and highly fragrant, white, star-shaped flowers. The flowers are harvested at night in order to obtain the most intense aroma. In India guests are often welcomed with garlands of the flowers. Jasmine is popular as a flavouring for tea in China; and in Europe it is used medicinally. The plant is grown in many parts of the world, including the Middle East, China, North Africa, France and Italy.

APPLICATIONS AND EFFECTS

It has a strong, masculine scent and produces feelings of optimism, euphoria and confidence.

Skin: Dry, greasy, irritated or sensitive skin (but see caution, below).

Circulatory and muscular systems: Muscular spasm, sprains.

Respiratory system: Catarrh, coughs, laryngitis, hoarseness.

Reproductive and excretory systems: PMS, painful periods; promotes labour and lactation.

Nervous system: Depression, nervous exhaustion.

Mental/emotional effects: This emotionally warming oil has the ability to unite the opposing factors within us. It is most useful at times when there is apathy, indifference, and coldness.

CAUTION: Generally safe to use, although some individuals may have an allergic reaction to it. It can give some people a headache and its narcotic quality may impede concentration.

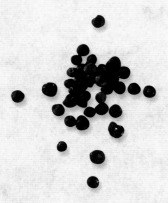

JUNIPER
Juniperus communis

This evergreen tree or shrub has fine, stiff, needle-like leaves of bluish-green and small flowers that are followed by tiny berries. The tree is native to Scandinavia, Siberia, Canada, northern Europe, and Asia. Its medicinal properties are known throughout the world. The Greeks, Romans, and Arabs valued its antiseptic properties, while the Mongolians used it to assist women in labour. More recently, juniper and rosemary have been burned to clear the air in French hospitals. In the Bible, Elijah sleeps under a juniper tree (Kings 1:19:4–5), connecting it with the ability to revive the spirits.

APPLICATIONS AND EFFECTS

Its most important use is as a detoxifier. Also particularly effective for cellulite, absence of menstrual periods, cystitis, water retention and painful periods.

Skin: Acne, dermatitis, eczema, haemorrhoids, toner for oily skin, wounds.

Circulatory and muscular systems: Toxic states generally, gout, arthritis, cramps, rheumatism.

Digestive system: Detoxifying.

Immune system: Colds, 'flu, coughs, purification of the blood, useful following infection.

Nervous system: Anxiety, nervous tension.

Mental/emotional effects: Strengthens the spirit and purifies the atmosphere. Can help in challenging situations and when overcome with feelings of regret for past actions.

CAUTION: Some people may find it irritating, and it is best avoided during pregnancy. Not to be used by people with kidney disease.

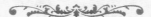

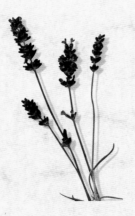

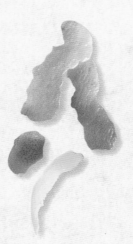

LAVENDER
Lavandula angustifolia/officinalis

Lavender has been the most popular essential oil for centuries. The plant is an easily recognized evergreen shrub with narrow, pale silver-green leaves and spikes of flowers ranging in colour from pink and white to pale or deep blue. It is widely cultivated in France, Bulgaria and England. Lavender was used by the Romans to bathe in and to cleanse wounds. In England it was commonly used to scent linen boxes, as an aid to controlling insects. Lavender water was the favourite perfume of Queen Henrietta Maria, wife of Charles I of England, and her partiality was responsible for it becoming popular and fashionable.

APPLICATIONS AND EFFECTS

Mellow, peaceful and the most versatile of all the essential oils. Particularly useful for burns, stress headaches and insomnia.

Skin: Sunburn, bruises, earache, insect bites, cuts.
Circulatory and muscular systems: Muscular aches and painful rheumatism.
Digestive system: Nausea, vomiting, flatulence, indigestion.
Reproductive and excretory systems: Painful and scanty periods.
Immune system: 'Flu, colds, myalgic encephalomyelitis (ME).
Nervous system: Stress headaches, insomnia, shock, vertigo.
Mental/emotional effects: Gently sedative, its balancing action makes it useful for panic states, or impatience and anger. Lavender cleanses both physically and spiritually. It aids in breaking bad habits and is soothing during a crisis.

LEMON
Citrus limonum

The lemon tree is native to Asia, although it now grows wild in the Mediterranean, particularly in Spain and Portugal. It is cultivated extensively in many parts of the world, including North and South America, Israel, Guinea, Cyprus, Sicily and Italy. The tree grows to only 2 m/6 ft in height; it is evergreen with small serrated oval leaves and highly fragrant pink or white flowers. The fruits ripen from green to yellow. The oil was used by the ancient Egyptians as an antidote to food poisoning, and to cure epidemics of fever. In most European countries it was regarded as a cure, but its main use was as a treatment for infectious disease.

APPLICATIONS AND EFFECTS

Fresh, strong and versatile, it harmonizes well and adds character. Particularly effective for arthritis, rheumatism, cellulite, nausea, diarrhoea and haemorrhoids.

Skin: Acne, brittle nails, boils, chilblains, greasy skin, cold sores, insect bites, mouth ulcers, spots, warts, verrucas, bruises.
Circulatory and muscular systems: Nosebleeds, congestion, poor circulation, muscular aches and pains.
Respiratory system: Throat infections, bronchitis, catarrh, sinusitis.
Digestive system: Indigestion, flatulence, heartburn, constipation.
Nervous system: Headaches, migraine.
Immune system: Colds, 'flu, fever, coughs, infections (chronic and recurrent), candida, allergies.
Mental/emotional effects: Can help refresh and clarify thought. Good for feelings of bitterness or resentment about life's injustices, and useful when someone is feeling touchy or when begrudging others' good fortune and success.

CAUTION: May sensitize the skin in some people. Use with caution when sunbathing as it may cause skin discoloration and rash.

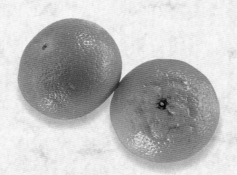

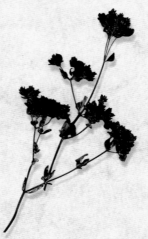

MANDARIN
Citrus reticulata

The fruit of the mandarin tree was the ancient and traditional gift to the mandarins of China, where the plant is a native species. It is an evergreen tree with shiny leaves, fragrant white flowers and juicy, edible fruit. The tree was introduced to Europe at the beginning of the nineteenth century, and some 40 years later into the United States. The Americans renamed the tree and fruit the tangerine, but the latter is in fact a larger and rounder fruit with a more yellow skin than the mandarin. The mandarin is grown in Italy, Spain, Algeria, Cyprus, Greece, the Middle East and Brazil.

APPLICATIONS AND EFFECTS

Refined, soft, cheerful, uplifting, sweet. Particularly effective for congested pores and oily skin, and fluid retention.

Skin: Acne, spots, stretch marks.

Circulatory and muscular systems: Helps to tone and improve the circulation.

Digestive system: Digestive problems, pain, flatulence, heartburn, nausea, hiccups.

Nervous system: Insomnia, restlessness, nervous tension.

Mental/emotional effects: This is a balancing oil that can be relaxing or a tonic, according to the individual's needs. It is good for dejected spirits and feelings of emotional emptiness, or the regretting of the passage of time and past losses. It is uplifting, and brings the message of happiness to children. It also helps adults make contact with their own inner child.

CAUTION: Generally safe to use but, like other citrus oils, it should be used with caution in the sun and under other sources of ultraviolet light.

MARJORAM
Origanum majorana

Marjoram is a small perennial plant with hairy stems and dark green, oval leaves. It is native to the Mediterranean region and North Africa, and was often planted in graveyards to bring peace to the departed spirits. The Latin name may be derived from *maior*, meaning "greater", not because there is a lesser variety, but in the sense of conferring longevity. The species name is derived from two Greek words, *oros* and *ganos*, which together mean "joy of the mountains". The herb is used extensively in cooking. The essential oil is extracted from the leaves; it has a very bitter taste and a refined fragrance.

APPLICATIONS AND EFFECTS

Gentle, warming and comforting. Particularly effective for constipation, flatulence, menstrual disorders, anxiety, tension, panic and insomnia.

Skin: Chilblains, bruises.

Circulatory and muscular systems: Arthritis, muscular aches and stiffness, rheumatism, sprains, strains.

Respiratory system: Bronchitis, coughs.

Digestive system: Colic.

Reproductive and excretory systems: PMS.

Immune system: Colds.

Nervous system: Headaches.

Mental/emotional effects: A sedative oil and aphrodisiac. Helpful in highly excitable states and may be useful for hyperactive children. Strengthens the mind and aids in confronting difficult issues such as recent grief.

CAUTION: Best avoided during pregnancy.

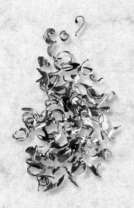

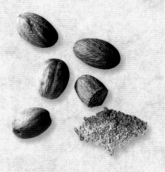

NEROLI
Citrus aurantium

The evergreen tree from which the essential oil is produced is native to China, where it was used by traditional Chinese herbalists. The expressed oil is produced in Israel, Cyprus, Brazil and North America. It is a less robust and smaller plant than the bitter orange variety and without the spiny branches or the heart-shaped leaves. The flowers were traditionally used in wedding bouquets to symbolize innocence and to secure love. Orange flower water features in Eastern European cookery and is an ingredient in eau-de-Cologne, which was very popular with those Victorian ladies frequently overcome with the "vapours". Neroli is one of the finest of the floral essences.

APPLICATIONS AND EFFECTS

Simple happiness; nourishing to the soul. Particularly effective for nervous diarrhoea and stress-related conditions.

Skin: Dull, oily, dry and sensitive skin, mouth ulcers, broken veins.
Circulatory and muscular systems: Palpitations, poor circulation.
Respiratory system: Bronchitis, chills.
Digestive system: Constipation, indigestion, flatulence, nausea.
Nervous system: Nervous tension, headaches and insomnia.
Immune system: Colds, 'flu.
Mental/emotional effects: Hypnotic and euphoric. Gives a feeling of peace; useful during times of anxiety, panic, hysteria or shock and fear. Invaluable for soothing when difficulties stem from a relationship. It can help in the development of self-esteem and self-love, comfort the sad, and bring people into contact with their feminine aspect.

CAUTION: The distilled oil is phototoxic, but the expressed oil is not. Generally safe to use although some individuals may get dermatitis.

NUTMEG
Myristica fragrans

Nutmeg and mace are most widely used as culinary spices both in the East and West. The fruit is like a small peach of which the nutmeg is the seed, contained in a bright red husk. Mace, the husk, is used independently as a milder spice than nutmeg. The tree is cultivated in Indonesia, Sri Lanka and the West Indies – particularly Grenada – and the oil is distilled in Europe and the United States. Nutmeg oil has been used in diverse ways, for example in Malaysia as a tonic for pregnant women, and in the manufacture of candles and soap. The Egyptians used it in embalming and in Italy it was an ingredient in incense, used to give protection against the plague.

APPLICATIONS AND EFFECTS

Particularly effective for muscular aches and pains, poor circulation, sluggish digestion, loss of appetite and the early stages of a cold.
Circulatory and muscular systems: Arthritis, gout, rheumatism.
Digestive system: Flatulence, indigestion, nausea, constipation.
Immune system: Bacterial infection, convalescence.
Nervous system: Nervous fatigue.
Mental/emotional effects: This oil is warming, stimulating and a euphoric. It can be comforting to those who find themselves physically and emotionally isolated, such as the elderly.

CAUTION: Use in moderation and with care during pregnancy.

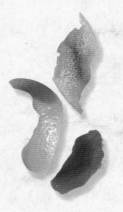

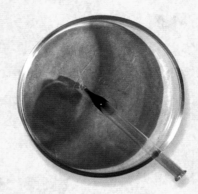

ORANGE
Citrus aurantium

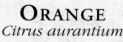

The essential oil called orange and the preserve, marmalade, come from the small, bitter fruit known as the Seville orange, which differs from the familiar, edible, sweet orange, *Citrus sinensis. C. aurantium* has shiny, dark green, oval leaves that are pale beneath; the smooth, grey-green branches have long, blunt spines and the small, white flowers are highly fragrant. The plant has become a symbol of both innocence and fertility. The Crusaders brought it back to Europe with them from North Africa and early missionaries introduced it into California. The United States is now one of the main producers of the oil. Because the oil oxidizes very quickly it cannot be kept for very long.

APPLICATIONS AND EFFECTS

Mellow, warming and soothing. Has similar properties to neroli and can be used in similar conditions.
Skin: Dull and oily complexions, mouth ulcers.
Circulatory and muscular systems: Muscular aches and pains, water retention, detoxifying.
Respiratory system: Bronchitis, chills.
Digestive system: Constipation, colic, indigestion (aids digestion of fats), diarrhoea, stimulates appetite.
Immune system: Colds, 'flu, fevers.
Nervous system: Nervous tension, insomnia due to anxiety.
Mental/emotional effects: Lifts gloomy thoughts and depression and encourages a positive outlook. Useful for replenishing cheerfulness. Revives the spirit when it is lacking in energy and relieves boredom. Quells "butterflies" in the stomach.

CAUTION: Generally safe to use, although, like other citrus oils, it increases the photosensitivity of the skin and can cause irritation under ultraviolet light, particularly from the sun. Occasionally causes dermatitis.

PALMAROSA
Cymbopogon martini

This herbaceous plant is native to India and Pakistan, but is cultivated in parts of Africa, in Indonesia, the Comoro Islands and Brazil. Palmarosa has fine, elegant stems and bears flowers on the tip of each stem. The oil is extracted from the leaves. At one time it was exported from the sub-continent and shipped from Bombay to the Red Sea ports. From there it was taken overland to Istanbul (then Constantinople) and to Bulgaria, where it was used to adulterate the highly prized rose oil known as attar of roses, gaining the name "Indian" or "Turkish" oil.

APPLICATIONS AND EFFECTS

Gentle and comforting. Particularly effective for skin inflammations, scars, weak digestion and headaches.
Skin: Acne, dermatitis, minor skin infections, scars, sores; all skin types.
Circulatory and muscular systems: Rheumatic conditions.
Respiratory system: Palpitations.
Digestive system: Intestinal infections.
Reproductive and excretory systems: Candida, cystitis.
Immune system: Myalgic encephalomyelitis (ME).
Nervous system: Nervous exhaustion.
Mental/emotional effects: This is a refreshing oil that can be an aid to spiritual healing. Its cooling quality is useful for anger, jealousy, irritability, hot-headedness and burning, passionate feelings.

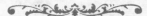
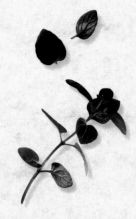

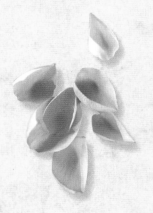

PEPPERMINT
Mentha piperita

Peppermint is a perennial herb that is cultivated throughout the world. White peppermint has green stems and leaves, the black variety has dark green, serrated leaves, purplish stems and reddish-violet flowers. Legend relates how Mentha, a nymph pursued by Hades, was trampled into the ground by Hades' jealous wife, Persephone. Out of compassion for her treatment, Hades transformed Mentha into the herb. Peppermint's medicinal qualities were widely appreciated by the ancient Egyptians, Chinese and Indians. The Romans used to crown themselves with peppermint wreaths during feasts, in order to take advantage of its detoxifying effects.

APPLICATIONS AND EFFECTS

Particularly useful for muscular aches and pains, sore feet, headache, indigestion and flatulence, stomach cramps, nausea, colds, fevers.
Skin: Acne, dermatitis, toothache.
Circulatory and muscular systems: Palpitations.
Respiratory system: Bronchitis.
Digestive system: Morning and travel sickness, bad breath.
Immune system: 'Flu, sinusitis.
Mental/emotional effects: Useful for mental fatigue and as an aid to clear thinking. Helpful for anger or hysteria, nervous trembling, shyness and hyper-sensitivity. Overcomes feelings of inferiority by dispelling pride. Associated with cleanliness and the wish to live ethically.

CAUTION: Can be a slight irritant for sensitive skins. May counteract the effects of homeopathic remedies, and suppress milk flow in breast-feeding mothers. Too much in the evenings may cause disturbed sleep patterns.

ROSE
Rosa × *damascena trigintipetala*

The fresh rose petals used to produce the essential oil are harvested early in the morning just after the dew has settled, and distilled immediately to maximize the yield. The finest oil – the famous and extremely expensive attar of roses – comes from an area in Bulgaria, lying halfway between Sofia and the Black Sea, known as the Valley of Roses. Other roses used in the production of rose oil include *Rosa centifolia*, or the Provence rose. These are also cultivated in Grasse, the centre of the perfume industry in the South of France.

APPLICATIONS AND EFFECTS

Promotes a feeling of well-being and the development of tolerance. Particularly effective for mature skin and stomach upsets with an emotional origin.
Skin: Broken veins, conjunctivitis, dry skin, eczema, sensitive skin.
Circulatory and muscular systems: Palpitations, poor circulation.
Respiratory system: Coughs, allergies affecting the lungs.
Digestive system: Liver congestion (caused by a surplus of blood), nausea, constipation.
Reproductive and excretory systems: Irregular and painful periods.
Nervous system: Depression, insomnia, headache, nervous tension.
Mental/emotional effects: Loneliness, grief and past emotional trauma, such as repressed anger or problems in relationships, can all be helped by this euphoric oil. Useful when dealing with bitter feelings such as jealousy or smouldering anger. Helps people make a fresh start, as it is emotionally healing and cleansing.

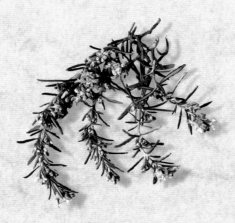

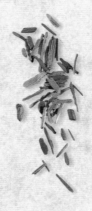

ROSEMARY
Rosmarinus officinalis

Rosemary is a shrubby evergreen bush cultivated in most parts of the world, but native to the Mediterranean region. It has scented, silver-grey, needle-like leaves and pale lilac or blue flowers, from which the oil is distilled. In ancient Greece it was burned in shrines, and in ancient Rome it was regarded as a symbol of regeneration. The Moors planted it around their orchards as an insect repellent and it was used in the Middle Ages as a fumigant to drive away evil spirits. More recently, the French used it as a disinfectant in hospital wards during epidemics.

APPLICATIONS AND EFFECTS

Vigorous, penetrating and stimulating. Particularly effective as a remedy for fluid retention and muscular pain.

Skin: Acne, dandruff, dermatitis, eczema, greasy hair, insect repellent.

Circulatory and muscular systems: Gout, palpitations, poor circulation, rheumatism.

Respiratory system: Bronchitis.

Digestive system: Flatulence, indigestion.

Reproductive and excretory systems: Painful menstrual periods.

Nervous system: Debility, headaches, high blood pressure, mental fatigue, nervous exhaustion.

Mental/emotional effects: It can be useful for mental fatigue or lethargy, poor memory or confusion. Rosemary strengthens the mind where there is weakness and exhaustion, and can be used when feeling apathetic or desiring to escape. It is a psychic protector for both individuals and places.

CAUTION: Should be avoided in pregnancy and by epileptics, and used with caution by those with sensitive skins.

SANDALWOOD
Santalum album

Sandalwood has a persistent, sensuous perfume and is one of the oldest-known scented materials, with perhaps as many as 4000 years of uninter-rupted use. The essential oil of *Santalum album* is distilled from the heart-wood of 30- to 60-year-old evergreen trees growing in Mysore, India. Because the wood is resistant to ant infestation, it was used in the construction of both furniture and buildings, a use that eventually resulted in near extinction of the species. Export of the wood is now illegal and all trees are owned by the Indian government. Oils originating from countries other than India are far inferior in quality.

APPLICATIONS AND EFFECTS

Gentle and sedative. Particularly effective for acne, dry and oily skins, persistent coughs, cystitis, stress and fear.

Skin: Dehydrated, cracked or chapped skin, barber's rash, itching, inflammation, dry eczema, boils, cuts and wounds.

Respiratory system: Bronchitis, catarrh, dry coughs, laryngitis, sore throat.

Immune system: Immune system booster for persistent conditions.

Nervous system: Depression, insomnia, diarrhoea caused by nervous conditions, paranoia; a sensual stimulant.

Mental/emotional effects: Can help encourage self-expression and boost lack of confidence. Brings peace and acceptance, and is therefore useful for grieving, helping the individual cut their ties with the past. Creates a balance for possessive and manipulative people who have difficulty in forgiving. Quietens mental chatter while meditating, allowing deeper meditative states to be reached; useful for healing and self-healing.

CAUTION: May sometimes cause contact dermatitis.

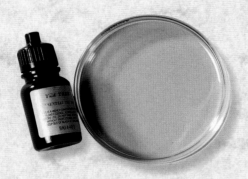

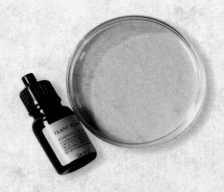

TEA TREE
Melaleuca alternifolia

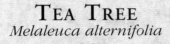

The tea tree is native to Australia, and is cultivated for its oil along the coast of New South Wales. It has narrow leaves and bears yellow or purple flowers. The essential oil is one of only a few that have been extensively studied. The results revealed that tea tree oil is active against all types of infectious organisms: bacteria, fungi and viruses. It is also a very powerful immune stimulant, increasing the body's ability to respond to these organisms. The oil was a component of tropical first-aid kits during the Second World War, but as antibiotics were developed it was dropped from use, only to be rediscovered as aromatherapy has gained in popularity.

APPLICATIONS AND EFFECTS
Particularly effective in fighting infectious organisms.
Skin: Abscess, acne, athlete's foot, blisters, cold sores, dandruff, dry scalp, insect bites, rashes (nappy rash), spots, verrucas, warts, infected wounds.
Respiratory system: Bronchitis, catarrh, coughs, sinusitis, throat infections, ear infections.
Reproductive and excretory systems: Thrush, cystitis.
Immune system: Colds, fevers, 'flu, infectious diseases including chicken-pox, systemic candida, mouth ulcers, myalgic encephalomyelitis (ME), post-operative shock, reducing the risk of infection, boosting the immune system in convalescence.
Nervous system: The oil is vigorous and revitalizing, and is particularly useful after shock. It is also very refreshing.

CAUTION: Some individuals may develop a sensitivity to it.

YLANG YLANG
Cananga odorata

The name ylang ylang means "flower of flowers", and the very fragrant plant is sometimes called "poor man's jasmine". The source of this essential oil is a beautiful evergreen tree native to Madagascar and the Philippines. It is now cultivated in several parts of the world, including Sumatra, Java and the Comoros. The oil comes from the tree's delicate yellow flowers, which have a very sweet scent reminiscent of almonds and jasmine. Many different qualities of oil are available; the finest is said to come from the flowers of trees grown in Réunion and picked in early morning at the beginning of summer. In Indonesia the voluptuously fragrant flowers are ceremonially scattered on the beds of newly married couples. The essential oil is widely used in perfumes and other aromatic products.

APPLICATIONS AND EFFECTS
Particularly effective for accelerated breathing and palpitations, insomnia and bowel infections.
Skin: Combination skin.
Circulatory and muscular systems: High blood pressure.
Digestive system: Gastro-enteritis.
Nervous system: Depression, anxiety.
Mental/emotional effects: This exotic, luxurious oil creates a feeling of peace and dispels anger, especially anger born of frustration. Its voluptuous nature is reassuring and builds confidence.

CAUTION: Some people may feel headachy or nauseous after using the oil, especially if it is used in concentrated form.

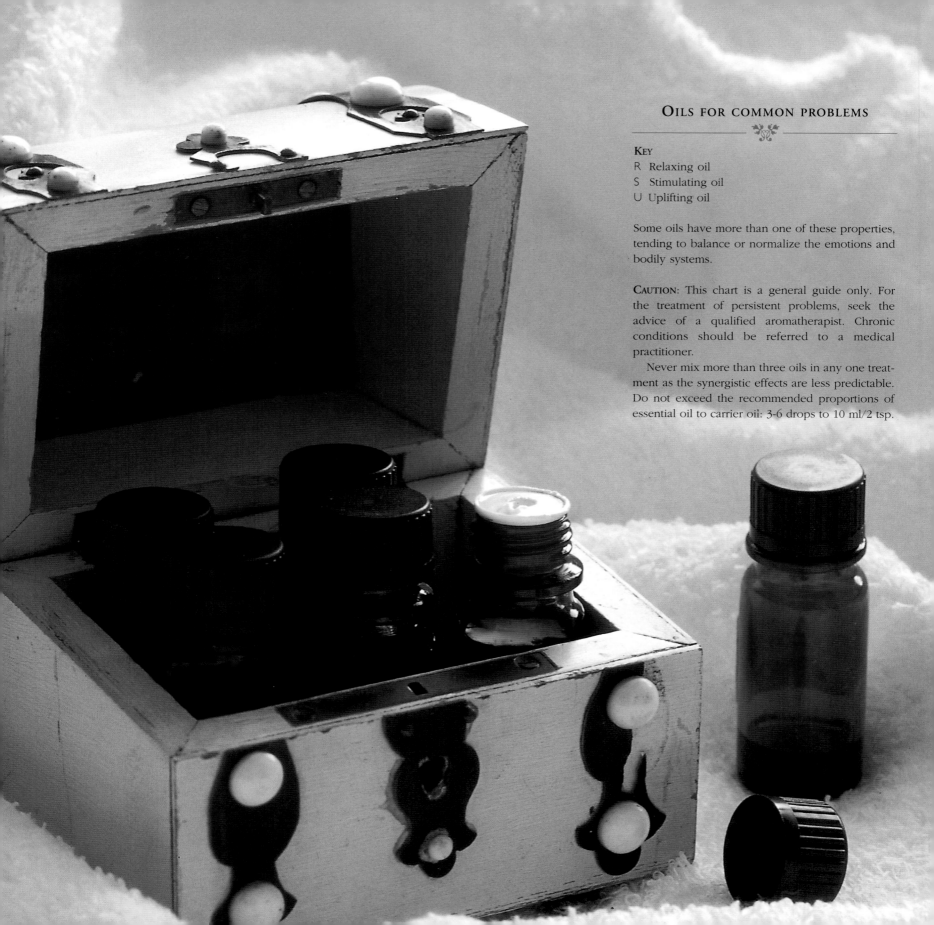

OILS FOR COMMON PROBLEMS

KEY

R Relaxing oil
S Stimulating oil
U Uplifting oil

Some oils have more than one of these properties, tending to balance or normalize the emotions and bodily systems.

CAUTION: This chart is a general guide only. For the treatment of persistent problems, seek the advice of a qualified aromatherapist. Chronic conditions should be referred to a medical practitioner.

Never mix more than three oils in any one treatment as the synergistic effects are less predictable. Do not exceed the recommended proportions of essential oil to carrier oil: 3-6 drops to 10 ml/2 tsp.

Oil		Acne	Anxiety	Arthritis	Athlete's Foot	Blood pressure: High	Blood pressure: Low	Body odour	Bronchitis	Cellulite	Colds/chills	Constipation	Cystitis	Dandruff	Depression	Diarrhoea	Eczema	Fainting	Flatulence	Haemorrhoids	Hayfever	Headaches	Hormonal regulation	Indigestion	Influenza	Insomnia	Menopausal problems	Menstrual problems (general)	Irregular periods	Painful periods	Mental fatigue	Muscular aches	Nausea	Obesity	Pre-menstrual syndrome	Rheumatism	Sexual problems	Sinusitis	Stress	Throat infections	Travel sickness	Varicose veins	Warts	Water Retention
Basil	R, U		✿						✿		✿				✿			✿	✿			✿		✿	✿			✿					✿		✿									
Bay	R			✿				✿	✿																											✿								
Benzoin	S			✿					✿		✿		✿																															
Bergamot	R, U	✿	✿										✿		✿				✿																					✿				
Black Pepper	S			✿							✿	✿				✿			✿													✿	✿			✿								
Cedarwood	R	✿							✿					✿	✿		✿									✿											✿							
Chamomile	R	✿	✿	✿								✿			✿	✿	✿		✿	✿	✿	✿	✿	✿		✿						✿	✿		✿	✿			✿					
Cinnamon	R						✿				✿					✿								✿	✿							✿				✿								
Comfrey	R				✿												✿										✿			✿		✿												
Cypress	R		✿					✿		✿			✿			✿			✿				✿		✿		✿	✿				✿	✿		✿							✿		✿
Eucalyptus	S	✿		✿					✿		✿		✿			✿				✿	✿	✿			✿							✿				✿		✿		✿			✿	
Fennel	S											✿							✿								✿						✿	✿										
Frankincense	R										✿														✿															✿				
Geranium	R, U		✿											✿			✿						✿												✿	✿			✿					✿
Ginger	U										✿					✿			✿					✿				✿				✿	✿			✿		✿			✿			
Grapefruit	U	✿																													✿							✿						✿
Hyssop	R, S				✿				✿		✿					✿			✿						✿											✿								
Jasmine	R	✿	✿												✿															✿							✿		✿					
Juniper	R, U	✿	✿							✿			✿	✿		✿	✿		✿	✿					✿	✿		✿				✿		✿		✿						✿		✿
Lavender	R, U	✿	✿	✿	✿			✿	✿		✿				✿		✿	✿	✿			✿			✿	✿		✿				✿	✿		✿	✿		✿	✿	✿	✿	✿	✿	✿
Lemon	S	✿		✿							✿														✿									✿						✿		✿	✿	
Lemongrass	S	✿			✿			✿									✿																						✿		✿	✿		
Mandarin	U																		✿							✿						✿												
Marjoram	R		✿	✿	✿				✿			✿										✿				✿						✿				✿			✿					
Melissa	R, U		✿	✿	✿																	✿						✿																
Myrrh	S								✿		✿					✿	✿		✿																					✿				
Neroli	R		✿					✿									✿										✿	✿							✿		✿	✿						
Nutmeg	S			✿							✿	✿							✿													✿	✿											
Orange	U		✿			✿						✿			✿												✿	✿																
Palmarosa	R	✿											✿																							✿								
Parsley	S			✿									✿																															✿
Patchouli	R	✿	✿		✿					✿				✿	✿		✿																✿				✿		✿					
Peppermint	S							✿	✿		✿					✿		✿	✿			✿		✿	✿								✿					✿		✿	✿	✿	✿	
Pine	S			✿					✿		✿		✿												✿							✿				✿		✿						✿
Rose	R		✿	✿											✿						✿		✿				✿	✿	✿	✿					✿		✿		✿					
Rosemary	S						✿				✿			✿	✿				✿			✿		✿							✿	✿		✿		✿						✿		✿
Sage	S			✿					✿																		✿					✿				✿				✿				✿
Clary Sage	R, S		✿		✿										✿				✿				✿				✿	✿	✿	✿					✿		✿		✿	✿				
Sandalwood	R	✿	✿						✿		✿		✿		✿		✿		✿								✿						✿				✿		✿	✿				
Tea Tree	S				✿						✿			✿											✿															✿			✿	
Thyme	S		✿	✿					✿										✿						✿								✿	✿	✿	✿				✿				✿
Ylang Ylang	R		✿			✿									✿																						✿		✿					

CARRIER OILS

Vegetable carrier oils are more than just vehicles for essential oils, as they often have health-giving qualities of their own. Choosing the appropriate carrier oil will add considerably to the dynamic nature of an aromatherapy massage and can have specific benefits, such as helping to guard against heart disease or inflammatory diseases such as arthritis.

Vegetable oils are made up of essential fatty acids and contain the soluble vitamins A, D and E. Some vegetable oils also contain large amounts of gamma linoleic acid (GLA), used in the treatment of PMS. The fatty-acid compounds help to reduce blood cholesterol levels and strengthen cell membranes, thereby slowing down the formation of fine lines and wrinkles by helping the body to resist attack by free radicals.

Always use a cold-pressed, unrefined certified organic vegetable oil for the dilution of essential oils. The darker the colour and stronger the odour, the less refined the oil, so it will be rich in health-giving properties. Once the bottle is opened, keep it in the fridge.

Experiment with different types of carrier oil. Try adding a teaspoonful of a second vegetable oil to the base oil, as well as the essential oils, for a highly personal mixture. Remember that the weather affects the skin, and central heating and cold wind will cause it to dry out. These variations can be accommodated by changing the exotic vegetable oils used to enrich each blend.

Almond oil

A good source of vitamin D. It is suitable for all skin types, especially dry or irritated skin.

Avocado oil

This oil is easily absorbed into the deep tissues and is therefore excellent for mature skin. It can help to relieve the dryness and itching of psoriasis and eczema. Although it blends well with others, it has a distinctive fruity smell, so use it with essential oils with complementary fragrances.

Borage oil

One of the richest sources of GLA, it is useful for the relief of eczema and psoriasis, as well as for the symptoms of PMS.

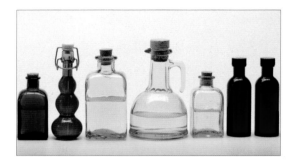

Store carrier oils carefully to ensure their freshness.

Carrot oil

A valuable source of beta carotene, carrot oil is useful for healing scar tissue and soothing acne and irritated skin.

Evening primrose oil

A rich source of GLA, useful for the relief of eczema, psoriasis, dry skin, PMS and tender breasts. It is also suitable for face treatments, but as it is quite a sticky oil it should be mixed with a lighter oil, such as grapeseed, soya, peanut or peachnut, for this purpose.

Grapeseed oil

A non-greasy oil which suits most skin types. It is most readily available in a refined state, so it is best to mix it with almond oil to enrich the blend.

Hazelnut oil

Hazelnut oil has unusual astringent qualities that are valuable for oily and combination skins.

Jojoba oil

Because it is rich in vitamin E, jojoba oil is excellent for sensitive or oily complexions, but is also good for all skin types and penetrates more easily than other oils. It contains bactericidal properties, making it a useful oil for the treatment of acne.

Olive oil

Olive oil is too sticky for massage, but a good addition to a blend for mature or dry skin.

Peachnut oil

A fine oil rich in vitamin E and good for delicate skin. It encourages elasticity and suppleness, and is particularly suitable for face massage.

Peanut oil

Highly nutritious in its unrefined state, but this is rarely available. In its refined form it makes a good carrier oil for massage purposes, but it is helpful to enrich it with a more nutritious oil.

Safflower oil

This oil has a light texture and penetrates the skin well. It is cheap and readily available in an unrefined state, making it a useful base for a blend.

Sesame oil

When made from untoasted seeds, sesame oil is good for skin conditions. It has sun screening properties and is used in suncare preparations.

Sunflower oil

Sunflower is a light oil rich in vitamins and minerals. It can be enriched by adding more exotic oils.

Walnut oil

Contains small amounts of GLA, and has a pleasant, nutty aroma.

Wheat germ oil

Rich in vitamin E and useful for dry and mature skin. It is well known for its ability to heal scar tissue, smooth stretch marks and soothe burns. As it is too sticky to use on its own as a massage oil, add small amounts of it to a lighter oil, but do not use on people with wheat intolerance.

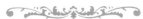

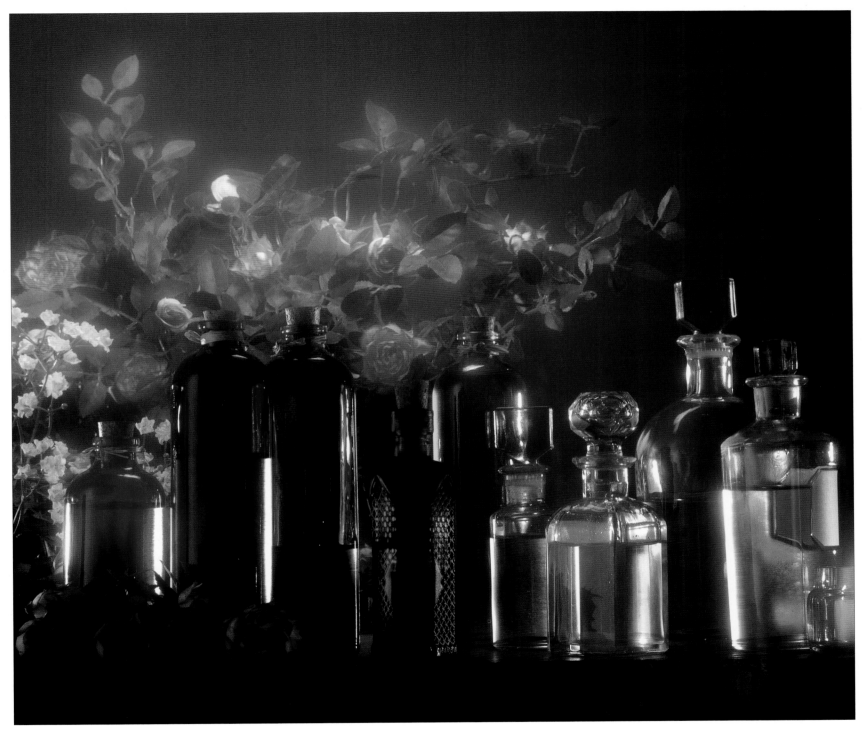

Carrier oils can be enriched with more exotic vegetable oils to create blends to suit specific skin types.

BLENDING AND STORING ESSENTIAL OILS

When essential oils are used for aromatherapy, different oils can be combined to increase their therapeutic effect.
As you become more practised in the art of blending you will begin to develop a nose for compatibility, in much the
same way as a perfumer blends scents, and you will be able to judge the best blend for your requirements by its aroma.
Once you have mixed your oils, store them carefully or use them immediately, as essential oils evaporate quickly.

Blending oils enables you to alleviate various physical and emotional symptoms in a single treatment, and while the combination of therapeutic properties is of prime importance, the value of fragrance should also be taken into account – no one enjoys taking unpleasant medicine, so don't underestimate the beneficial effects of a pleasing and sweet-smelling result when mixing your oils.

When blending oils for aromatherapy massage, the ratio of essential oil to carrier oil may vary, but as a general rule, up to 5 drops of essential oil in 10 ml/2 tsp carrier oil is enough for a body massage. This gives the recommended dilution for most massage purposes. However, if you are using oils for purely emotional problems, half the number of drops can be equally effective, while physical symptoms sometimes respond better to a higher percentage.

SYNERGY

When essential oils are blended, a chemical reaction occurs and the oils combine as a new compound. For example, when lavender is added to bergamot the sedative qualities of bergamot are increased; but if lemon is added to bergamot then its uplifting, refreshing aspect is enhanced. This process is known as synergy. Using this principle, oils can be blended so that they treat a person's emotional and physical needs at the same time. The blend can also be modified from treatment to treatment, depending on the time of day or the person's mood (for example, changing the balance of the blend, or substituting a different oil for one in the basic blend, can raise someone's spirits if they are low).

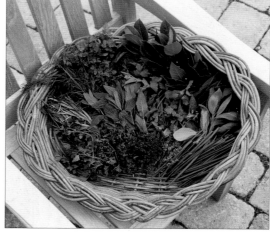

The natural aromas of essential oils blend as harmoniously as the plants from which they are distilled.

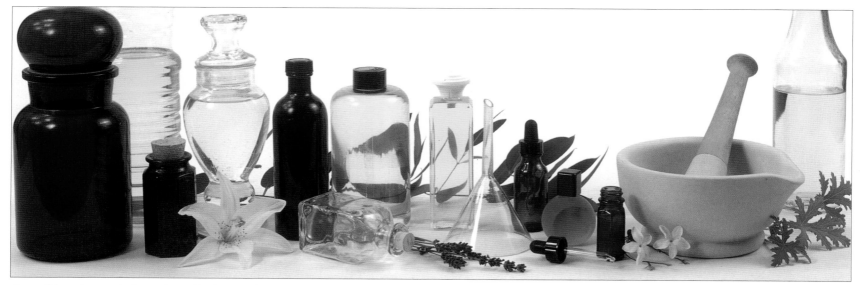

Be careful to mix enough of your chosen blend to complete a massage.

TOP, MIDDLE AND BASE NOTES

Essential oils are categorized by what are known as top, middle and base "notes". This is the way perfumers categorize scents, using different combinations of notes to create the balanced character of a new perfume. A good blend combines an oil from each category, and each oil is classified according to its dominant characteristic. You will eventually develop your own nose for which oils relate to each note. In general the fresh, herbaceous oils such as lemon, eucalyptus or tea tree are good top notes. The floral oils and some herb oils, such as lavender, geranium, chamomile and peppermint, make up the majority of the middle notes. The woody, resinous oils such as frankincense and sandalwood form the base notes. There are, however, some exceptions: rose and jasmine are unusually heady fragrances and although they are floral oils they are usually considered to be base notes.

Because they evaporate quickly, most blends should contain a higher percentage of top-note oil to each middle-note and base-note oil. For example, a well-balanced blend might be made up from 3 drops of orange (top note), 2 drops each of clary sage and geranium (both middle notes) and 2 drops of cedarwood (base note).

Top notes: fresh, light and immediately detectable because of their high evaporation rate.

Middle notes: the heart of the mixture, perceptible immediately after the top notes when smelling the blend for the first time.

Base notes: rich, heavy odours that linger and emerge fully only after more prolonged exposure to the blend.

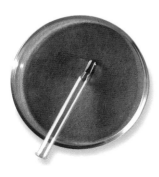

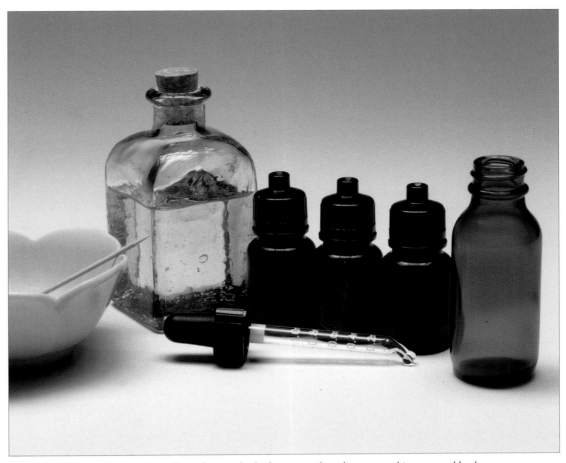

It is easier to predict the synergistic effects of essential oils if not more than three are used in any one blend.

STORAGE OF ESSENTIAL OILS

Essential oils last for a relatively long time if a few simple precautions are taken. They should always be bought in dark-coloured glass bottles with a stopper that automatically dispenses them a drop at a time. Keep the lid firmly closed to prevent evaporation, and store them in a cool place out of direct sunlight and away from direct heat. The citrus oils tend to go off more quickly than other oils, so it is a good idea to buy them in small quantities as you need them. It is easy to tell if an oil has deteriorated: it will become cloudy and give off a distinctly unpleasant odour. Always keep all essential oils out of the reach of children.

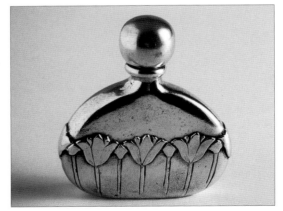

Store blended oils in tightly stoppered bottles, away from bright light.

AROMATHERAPY BLENDS FOR EVERYDAY WELL-BEING

As you become familiar with the aromas and properties of essential oils, you will want to experiment with blends that especially suit you. One of the delights of aromatherapy is the blending together of oils for an enhanced therapeutic effect, making a new fragrance to soothe the senses at the same time.

Throughout this book you will find recipes for well-balanced blends designed to help with specific problems. However, the sense of smell is very individual, so if you find that you do not like a particular combination, try something else, always bearing in mind the actions of the oils and the recommended dilution rates. Let your nose tell you if a blend is harmonious, but above all if you enjoy its aroma.

Here are some suggestions to guide you to the oils that will help you recover from the strains of everyday life, or enhance your mood on happy occasions. Choose up to three of the suggested essential oils, mixing them with a carrier oil, to make your own blends.

A BLEND TO AID RELAXATION

Relaxation is particularly important following a stressful day at work. Choose up to three oils from this list: bergamot, German chamomile, clary sage, lavender, rosewood or sandalwood. To add an uplifting note, choose one of the other citrus oils, which will produce a blend that is relaxing and uplifting at the same time.

A BLEND TO DISPEL GLOOM

When everything seems grey, a blend of some of the invigorating oils could help turn the day around from one of gloom and despair to a more energetic one. Try a blend of up to three of the following oils to stimulate and cleanse the system and make you feel more lively: black pepper, cypress, eucalyptus, fennel, ginger, grapefruit, jasmine, juniper, lemon, nutmeg, peppermint, rosemary or tea tree.

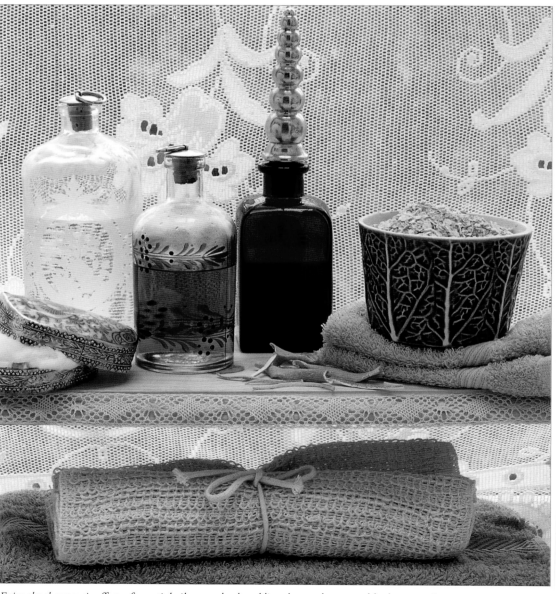

Enjoy the therapeutic effects of essential oils every day by adding them to beauty and bath preparations.

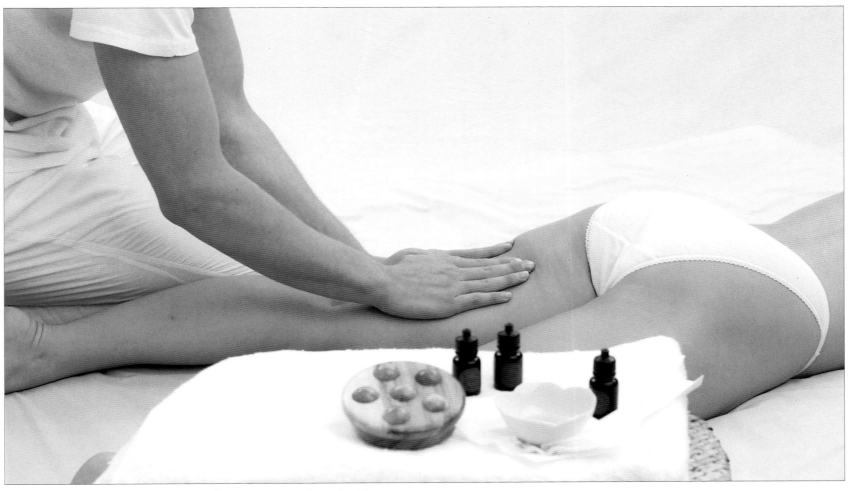

An aromatherapy massage is an ideal way to relieve tension or stimulate a sluggish system.

A BLEND FOR STIFF MUSCLES

Everyone can suffer from minor muscular aches and pains from time to time. They may be brought on by unusual physical exercise – from gardening or dancing to sporting activities – or simply by sitting or standing too long in an uncomfortable position. At such times the warming oils that bring blood back into the aching muscles are the most helpful. Choose from the following list: benzoin, black pepper, clary sage, eucalyptus, ginger, grapefruit, jasmine, juniper, lavender, lemon, marjoram, nutmeg, orange, peppermint or rosemary.

A REMEDY TO SOOTHE THE SKIN AFTER SUNBATHING

Prolonged sunbathing, particularly in the middle and hottest part of the day, can have a devastating effect on the skin. It encourages premature ageing and can be very painful. Prevention is, of course, better than cure, but if you are feeling tender and providing the skin is not actually burnt and broken, a gentle massage with a soothing oil is very comforting and moisturizing. Use rose and chamomile essential oils, and include some wheat germ oil in the blend which will also help to heal the skin.

A REMEDY FOR OVER-INDULGENCE

If you have had too much to drink, try to drink several glasses of water before sleeping, to help alleviate the dehydration caused by an excess of alcohol. Drink plenty of water and orange juice at breakfast to help speed up detoxification and, if you can, eat some wholemeal toast with a yeast spread. A blend of up to three of the following oils may help restore your system to normal good health after eating or drinking too much: black pepper, fennel, geranium, ginger, juniper, orange, peppermint.

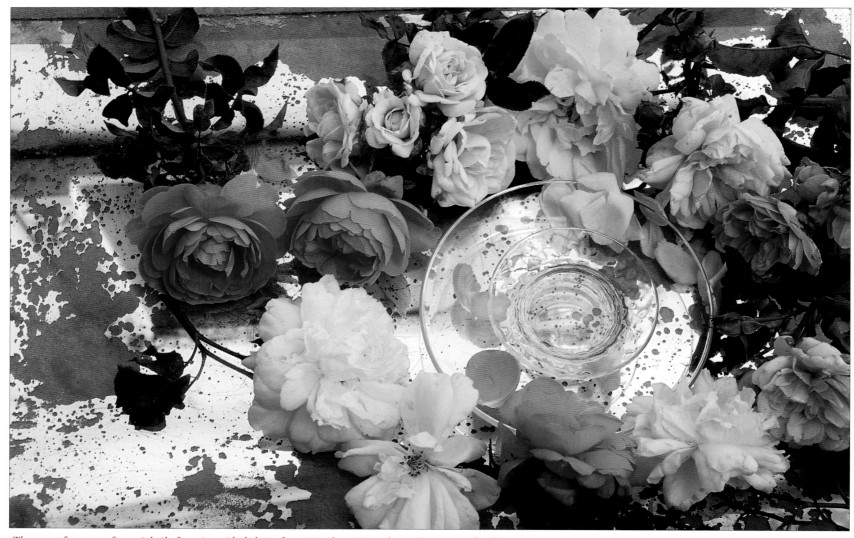

The warm fragrance of essential oil of rose is an ideal choice for raising the spirits and restoring a sense of well-being.

ESSENTIAL OILS FOR TRAVELLERS

If travelling is a source of anxiety for you, or if you suffer from travel sickness, essential oils can help to calm both the mind and the stomach. The simplest way to use them when you are travelling is to put a couple of drops on to a tissue or handkerchief and smell them frequently during the journey. Useful oils for this purpose are peppermint, mandarin or neroli.

A BLEND FOR RAISING THE SPIRITS

For the days when the ordinary activities of life seem too difficult, there are a number of oils that can help raise the spirits: benzoin, bergamot, cedarwood, clary sage, frankincense, geranium, grapefruit, jasmine, mandarin, nutmeg, orange, rose, rosewood or ylang ylang. A blend of up to three essential oils from this list can give you back your usual zest for life.

A BLEND TO BRING WARMTH AND COMFORT

After struggling with bitter winds and the cold of winter, there are some warming and comforting essential oils that can be very nourishing when you are feeling emotionally, as well as physically, cold. Blend benzoin, ginger, orange and rosewood together and allow them to envelop you in their special aroma.

AN APHRODISIAC BLEND

In a long-term relationship the intimate physical bond between partners may weaken or cease to exist. A long illness, overwork or emotional crises can also contribute to a lack of sexual interest. At such times the non-sexual but loving touch of massage can play an important part in rediscovering the sexual intimacy that has been missing. Essential oils that may help are: black pepper, cedarwood, clary sage, fennel, frankincense, ginger, jasmine, rose and sandalwood. Bear in mind that this is an area where it is especially important to take into account both partners' personal preferences for fragrance.

A NUPTIAL BLEND

There is only one blend to choose before a wedding: jasmine and rose, respectively the king and queen of fragrances, and neroli, to calm the nerves. This luxurious blend will bring the essence of calm to the beginning of married life.

A BLEND TO INSTIL PEACEFULNESS

Frankincense, sandalwood, neroli and ylang ylang blend together to create a rich perfume of peace. This blend can help recreate feelings of tranquillity and reduce feelings of fragmentation. It can be valuable in helping to reconnect you to your strong inner core and regain peace in your life.

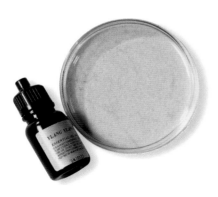

BLENDING ESSENTIAL OILS

Before you begin, wash and dry your hands and make sure that all your utensils are clean and dry. Have your essential oils at the ready, but leave the lids on the bottles until they are required.

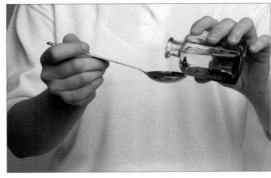

1 Carefully measure out 10 ml/2 tsp of your chosen vegetable oil.

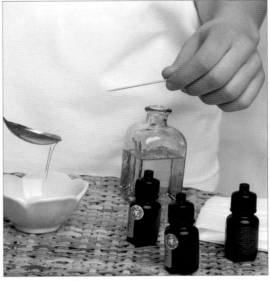

2 Gently pour the measured vegetable oil into your blending bowl.

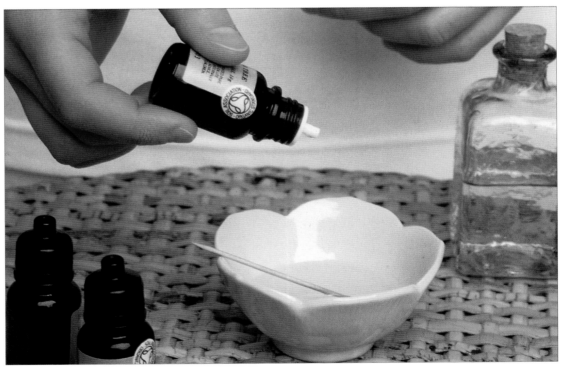

3 Add the first essential oil a drop at a time. Add the remaining oils a drop at a time, up to a maximum of 6 drops, and mix gently with a clean, dry cocktail stick or toothpick, to blend. Rub a little of the blend in your hands to test the fragrance.

USING ESSENTIAL OILS

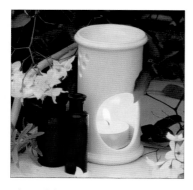

You can soak and splash in them, feed your skin, sensually smooth them all over, or simply breathe in their wonderful aromas. The pleasure and versatility of aromatic oils make them one of nature's kindest gifts. Essential oils contain the active ingredients of a plant in a highly concentrated and potent form. They therefore need to be treated with care and should never be applied directly to the skin undiluted. Massage, aromatic baths and inhalations are some of the most effective ways to use essential oils therapeutically, and are described on the following pages.

There are many ways of surrounding yourself with the uplifting or relaxing fragrances of the oils. Apart from vaporizers and sprays for scenting your home, you can experiment with your own blends of scents to create luxurious body oils, lotions and treatments for your hair. Wooden balls scented with aromatic oils will add fragrance to drawers used for storing clothes. Alternatively, you can scent paper drawer-liners and padded coat hangers with a few drops of essential oils such as melissa or bergamot, or cedarwood to deter moths. You can even deodorize your shoes with a drop of parsley or pine oil. Away from home, the most portable way of using essential oils is to sprinkle 3–4 drops on to a handkerchief and inhale the fragrance.

Add a few drops of an essential oil to hot water
to enjoy its unique aroma.

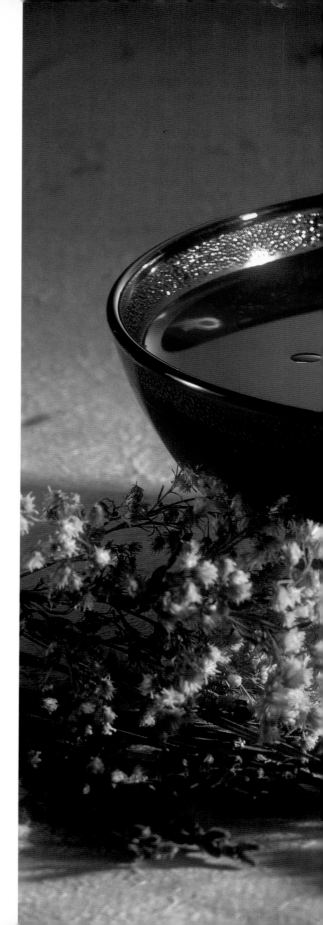

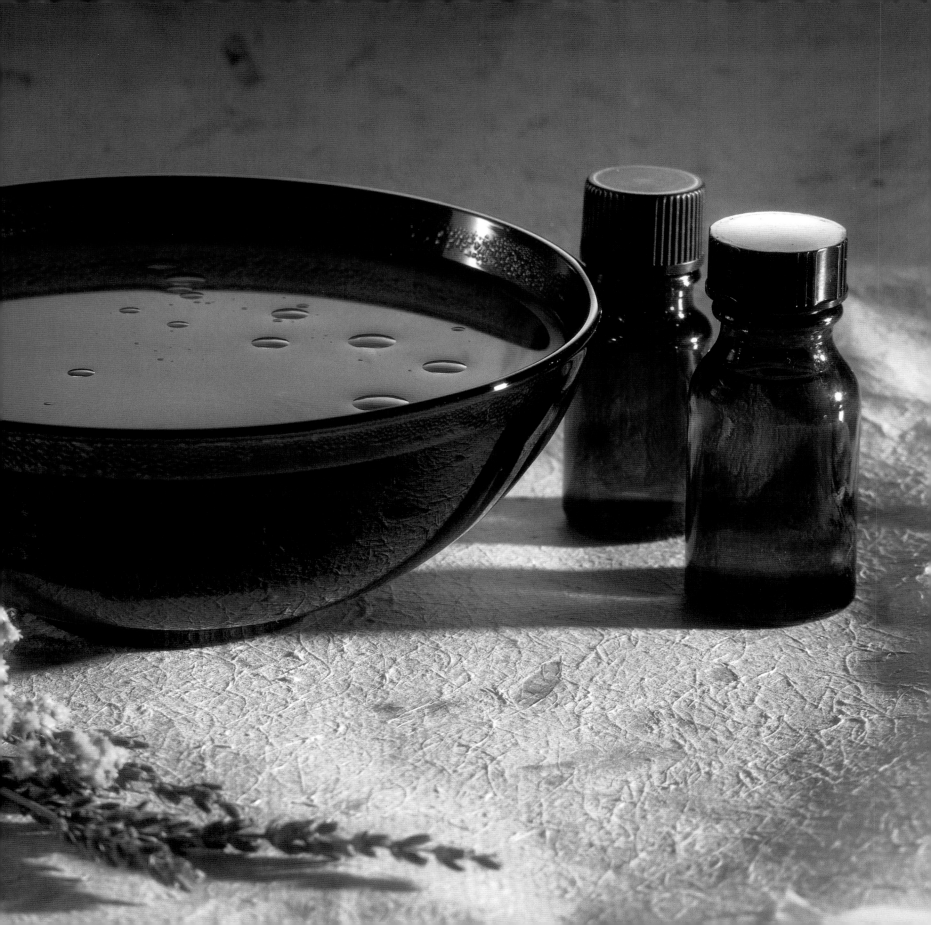

OILS IN THE AIR

A lingering smell, whether pleasant or not, is usually the first thing you notice when you enter a room, and it can strongly affect the way you feel. Fragrancing the home to delight the senses is an old tradition. For centuries the Chinese have suspended balls of jasmine flowers over the bed to clear the air and promote pleasant dreams, while bowls of potpourri, scented sachets and pomanders have a long history. Today, the methods of scenting a room are many and diverse. They can help prevent ill-health, balance the emotions and disguise unpleasant smells such as cigarette smoke or stale cooking odours.

LIVING ROOMS

Rose, geranium, orange and lavender are pleasing and uplifting scents for a room, used individually or blended together.

For an exotic, intimate atmosphere, use sandalwood or patchouli, or to unwind in the evening try geranium, lavender, sandalwood or ylang ylang.

Perfumes for parties

Clary sage or jasmine will create a heady, "feel-good" atmosphere for a party, or use orange, lemongrass or neroli for a lighter, fresher touch.

For a festive blend, choose from the spicier oils such as frankincense, cedarwood, sandalwood, cinnamon and orange.

STUDIES AND OFFICES

Useful oils for the workplace are basil, rosemary, bergamot, lemon and melissa. Bergamot and lemon are particularly antiseptic, and lemon has the added advantage of helping efficiency. Basil stimulates a tired brain and rosemary is a great aid to concentration. Rosemary is also helpful in relieving headaches. If you are feeling overwrought try clary sage or juniper, but watch the dosage as too much will cause sleepiness.

If you work in a large, open-plan space, fragrancing the whole area may not be a viable option. Sprinkle a few drops on a handkerchief or add a few drops of oil to a cup of hot water on your desk.

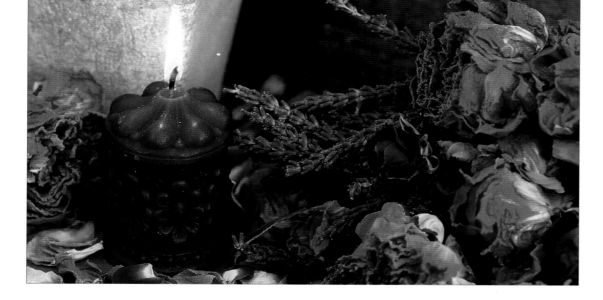

BEDROOMS

Whether to ensure a restful night's sleep or to turn your bedroom into a place of passion, fragrancing the bedroom just before bedtime will create an appropriate atmosphere. Rose, neroli and lavender are delightful all-purpose oils for the bedroom. Perfume your pillow with 2–3 drops of a relaxing oil to help you unwind, or one for insomnia if you have sleep problems. For a different mood, try an aphrodisiac like ylang ylang or be extravagant and use rose or jasmine, the two most luxurious and expensive essential oils.

Use lavender to freshen a musty spare room to make it welcoming for guests. Clear the atmosphere of a sick room with bergamot, eucalyptus or juniper.

KITCHENS AND BATHROOMS

Use tea tree, eucalyptus, melissa, lemongrass or the closely related citronella in a diffuser to keep insects at bay. Pine, lemon or tea tree can be used on a damp cloth to disinfect surfaces.

Vaporized molecules of any essential oil will neutralize airborne bacteria, but some – such as tea tree, bergamot, lemon, pine and lavender – are particularly antiseptic. Use these in a diffuser or room spray.

When you buy scented candles, make sure they have been made using natural essential oils.

DIFFUSING FRAGRANCES

Vaporizers come in many forms, but all work on the same principle. The reservoir is filled with water, to which are added drops of essential oil. The reservoir is then heated, causing the water to evaporate and the warm oil to release its perfume.

Make sure there is a suitable distance between the source of the heat and the reservoir for oil and water. This will reduce the risk of completely evaporating the water and thus burning the oil. The vaporizer should also be easy to clean ready for use with a different oil.

The simplest type of vaporizer has a candle as the heat source; a more efficient, but more expensive, type is the electric vaporizer, which is useful when you want to disperse oils for a long period of time without the necessity of frequent supervision. Some electric vaporizers have a silent fan that disperses the evaporating oils; others employ a heated ceramic dish. Either would be suitable for a child's or invalid's bedroom.

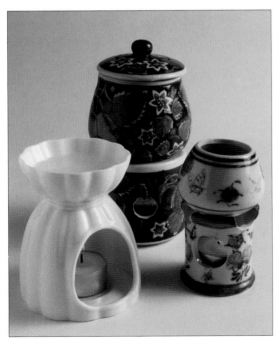

Simple vaporizers for essential oils disperse the fragrance quickly and effectively, and also make attractive ornaments.

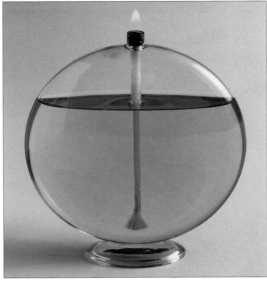

Add a few drops of essential oil to an oil lamp to scent a room.

How to use a vaporizer

Whenever you use a vaporizer of any kind, do make certain that you place it in a safe position, out of the reach of children and pets.

The number of drops of oil used in a burner depends on the size of the room: 2–3 drops for a small room, and as many as 6–10 for a larger one. It is better to use fewer drops and refresh the burner more frequently, rather than use too many and saturate the room with scent. Remember that your sensitivity to the scent will decrease, but this does not mean that the aroma is not still present and probably still quite strong.

Room sprays

To make a room spray, blend 10 drops of essential oil in 105 ml/7 tbsp water. 15 ml/1 tbsp vodka or pure alcohol added to the solution will act as a preservative, but this is optional. Shake well before filling a sprayer.

Humidifiers

You can add your favourite oil to the water of a humidifier or improvise by adding 5 drops of essential oil to a small bowl of water placed on top of a radiator.

Ring burners

Use the heat from light bulbs to release perfumed oils. Small ring burners, usually made of porcelain or aluminium, sit over the top of the bulb. Add a few drops of essential oil, and the heat from the bulb will gently vaporize the oil.

Wood fires

Sprinkle drops of cypress, cedarwood, pine or sandalwood over the logs to be used about an hour before lighting the fire and then burn them to release your favourite aroma.

Scented candles

Wax candles can be bought ready-impregnated with essential oils and are a delightful way of fragrancing a room. Or you can add a few drops of essential oil to an oil lamp for the same effect.

Potpourri

Add a few drops of an appropriate flowery or spicy essential oil to refresh tired potpourri.

To make a simmering potpourri, place a mixture of scented flowers and leaves (without any fixatives or additives) in a bowl of water and heat gently from below – a candle flame may well be sufficient. The aroma is not long-lasting, but is much stronger than that of dry potpourri. Add about 1 cupful of dried plant material to 1 litre/ 1¾ pints of water.

For a sleep-enhancing simmering potpourri, blend ½ cup lime flowers, ¼ cup chamomile flowers, 15 ml/1 tbsp sweet marjoram and 15 ml/ 1 tbsp lavender flowers. For a more refreshing, uplifting blend, try ½ cup lemon verbena leaves, ¼ cup jasmine flowers, 30 ml/2 tbsp lemon peel and 5 ml/1 tsp coriander seeds.

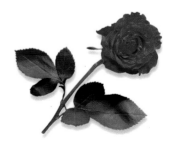

QUICK THERAPIES WITH ESSENTIAL OILS

In the middle of a busy day you may not have the time for a leisurely, relaxing bath or a full-body massage, but you can still benefit from the therapeutic effects of essential oils using these simple methods. The heat of the water will release the aromas of the oils immediately, so have everything ready for the treatment before you add them.

STEAM INHALATIONS

For problems like colds and sinus congestion, a steam inhalation warms and moistens the membranes, and the use of essential oils helps to open and relax the airways. Just boil a kettle, pour approximately ½ litre/1 pint hot water into a bowl, add the oils and inhale deeply. Use up to 5 drops for a strong medicinal effect, in cases of colds or chestiness, or just 2 drops for a gentler relaxing effect on the air passages.

RECOMMENDED ESSENTIAL OILS

A blend for nasal congestion:
For a stuffed-up feeling, maybe combined
with tiredness, use 3 drops eucalyptus
and 2 drops peppermint.

To ease a tight, tense chest:
For tension causing poor breathing,
relax the airways with 4 drops lavender
and 3 drops frankincense.

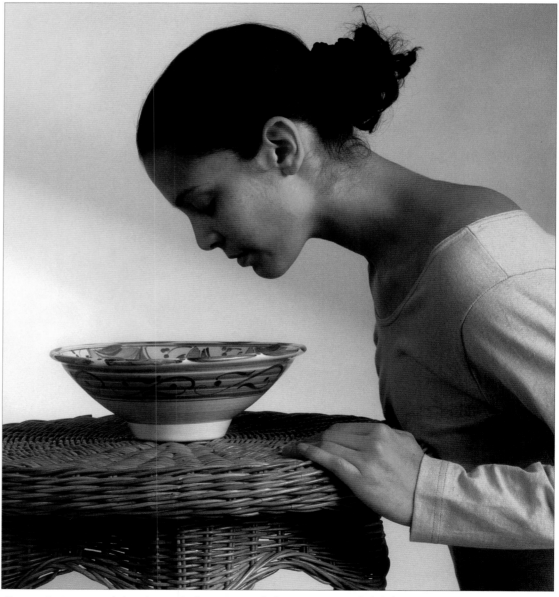

CAUTION: Do not overdo an inhalation, and if you have high blood pressure or asthma, seek medical advice before using steam.

For respiratory complaints in particular, steam inhalations are very helpful.

COMPRESSES

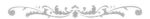

Hot or cold compresses are excellent ways to use oils for problems such as sprains and muscular aches. Cold compresses are suitable for use on acute injuries such as a strain or sprain, with swelling or bruising, though you should of course always seek medical advice in cases of serious injury. To make a cold compress, pour cold water over some ice in a bowl, add essential oils and soak a pad in the water before placing over the affected area and binding firmly in place.

For older injuries, with no swelling or inflammation, for chronic muscle pain and for arthritic or rheumatic pain, a hot compress may be more useful. For a hot compress: have the water as hot as you can comfortably bear. Pour it into a bowl, add the oils and use as above. Use 3–4 drops of essential oil in 250 ml/8 fl oz hot water (enough to fill an average-sized cereal bowl).

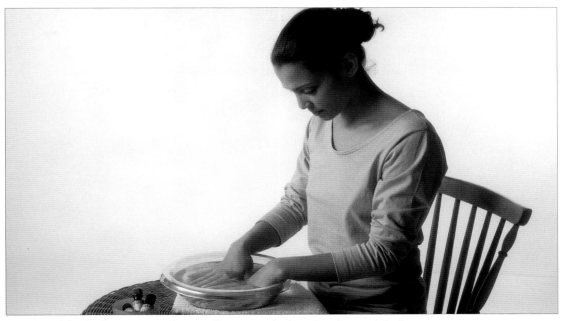

Hand and footbaths are a simple way of enjoying the benefits of essential oils.

RECOMMENDED ESSENTIAL OILS

A first aid remedy:
The ideal essential oil for a cold compress
is lavender, and this can be very useful
in many first aid situations.
Use 4 drops to a bowl of
iced water. Keep the pad on firmly
for at least 20 minutes, preferably
with the affected limb raised if there is
any swelling.

A blend for muscular pain:
For muscular aches and pains,
try using 2 drops each of rosemary and
marjoram in a bowl of hot water.
Apply the compress for
30 minutes.

HAND AND FOOTBATHS

A quick way to use essential oils is to make a hand or footbath; two-thirds fill a large bowl with hot water and add 3–4 drops of oils. The warmth of the water itself helps the blood vessels to dilate, and this can be very helpful in treating conditions such as tension headaches and migraines, when the blood vessels in the head are frequently engorged with blood. Try a foot or handbath at an early stage of a headache and see if you can drain away the excess stress.

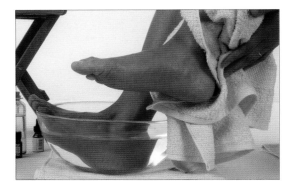

RECOMMENDED ESSENTIAL OILS

A blend to improve circulation:
For poor circulation and cold extremities, use
2 drops lavender and 2 drops marjoram oils.

Blends for aching muscles:
For tension and stiffness:
If stiffness is due to over-exertion, try a blend
of 2 drops rosemary and 2 drops pine.
To refresh hot, aching feet or hands:
Use a mixture of 2 drops peppermint and
2 drops lemon.

A footbath will not only relieve aching feet, but warm and invigorate the whole body.

THE AROMATIC BATH

A bath with essential oils is one of the simplest and most effective aromatherapy treatments. It can be stimulating or relaxing, depending on the temperature of the water and whether you choose oils with uplifting or calming properties. In the bath, the therapeutic action of the oils is twofold: they are absorbed through the skin, moisturizing the dermis and entering the circulatory system, and at the same time their aromas are inhaled, stimulating the brain and increasing your sense of well-being. An aromatic bath can detoxify the body and help with problems like cellulite, joint stiffness, general aches and pains, colds and headaches. It will also tone and condition the skin and relieve anxiety and tension.

RUNNING THE BATH

Bath temperature and the time spent in the tub are important. A cooler bath is more stimulating and warmer water relaxes. Very hot water is damaging, however: it causes blood vessels and capillaries to expand and increases the heart rate. You should particularly avoid hot water if you have varicose veins, haemorrhoids, high blood pressure or are pregnant. A 15–20 minute soak is long enough before skin cells over-hydrate, or swell with water.

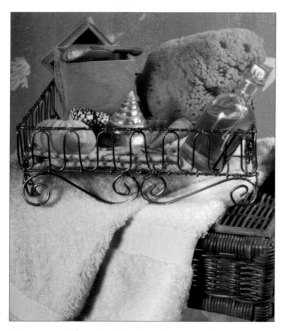

Use aromatherapy treatments to enhance your bathtime routine.

RECOMMENDED ESSENTIAL OILS

For stimulation:
Bergamot, cypress, eucalyptus, fennel, geranium, juniper, lavender, lemon, lemongrass, peppermint, pine, rosemary, thyme.

For relaxation:
Basil, cedarwood, chamomile, frankincense, hyssop, juniper, lavender, marjoram, melissa, neroli, patchouli, rose, sage, sandalwood, ylang ylang.

A morning blend:
For a refreshing, uplifting bath, try a blend of 3 drops bergamot and 2 drops geranium.

An evening blend:
To relax and unwind after a long day, make a blend of 3 drops lavender and 2 drops ylang ylang to add to your bath.

Bath oil formula (for three baths):
Mix a bath oil with a combination of up to three essential oils, up to 5 drops of each, in 15 ml/1 tbsp skin softening base oil. Choose oils with complementary effects. Use a third of the mixture for each bath.

OILS FOR THE BATH

Essential oils are the best way of making a bath both aromatic and therapeutic. They sink into the skin easily and at the same time impart their lovely herbal or floral fragrances.

You can add 5 drops of essential oil directly to the bath: they will float on the surface in a fine film and evaporate, giving you the full benefit of their aroma instantly.

If you want to absorb them more through the skin you can disperse them through the water by mixing with a base carrier oil such as sweet almond, apricot kernel, jojoba or evening primrose (these rich base oils all nourish and rejuvenate the skin in their own right, leaving it smooth and well moisturized).

THE STIMULATING BATH

The stimulating oils are best for the morning to get you started or to revive you at the end of a busy day before an evening out.

Keep the water fairly cool and use an invigorating bath mitt to rub down, enlivening the skin and stimulating the circulation. When you've soaked, rinse yourself with water as cold as you can bear, either by splashing directly from the tap or shower, or by adding more cold water to cool down your bath.

As you get out of the bath, either slap yourself dry to make the skin tingle or rub yourself vigorously with a towel.

THE RELAXING BATH

To calm yourself after a fraught day or to prepare yourself for a peaceful night's sleep, turn your bathroom into a private sanctuary. First, choose a time when you won't be interrupted by family or telephone calls. Keep the light in the room soft if possible, or use an eye mask or burn aromatic candles. Plants not only look good in the bathroom but also create an oxygenated atmosphere. Support your head with a bath pillow, close your eyes and inhale deeply. Concentrate on your breathing, empty your mind and let the oils soothe away the stresses and strains of the day. After a 15–20 minute soak, get out slowly and wrap yourself in a large, warm towel.

THE THERAPEUTIC BATH

Adding essential oils to a warm bath is also an effective way to exploit their physiological healing properties, particularly for skin problems as the warmth of the water will soften and relax the skin, allowing the oils to be absorbed readily.

RECOMMENDED ESSENTIAL OILS

For dermatitis:
Chamomile, hyssop, lavender.

For eczema:
Chamomile, geranium, hyssop, juniper, rosemary, myrrh.

For psoriasis:
Bergamot, chamomile, lavender.

For arthritis/rheumatism:
Chamomile, eucalyptus, juniper, lavender, rosemary, thyme.

A blend for aching muscles:
Add 3 drops marjoram and 2 drops chamomile essential oils to the bath.

SHOWERS AND COLD RINSES

Invigorating jets of water are ideal for getting the blood pumping and there's no need to forego the benefits of aromatic oils. Skin tends to be sluggish in the cold winter months but sloughing off dead top layers can help regenerate cells and allow moisturizers to be absorbed more easily. Showers are ideal for smoothing skin with exfoliating rubs using wet salt, a loofah or a friction mitt. Soften loofahs and mitts first in warm water. Soft bristle brushes can also help to get the circulation going with gentle massage on problem areas like hips and thighs. To keep brushes and mitts fresh, always rinse them and hang them up to dry.

Essential oils can be used under the shower: mix a base oil with invigorating essences, pour on to a clean face-cloth or sponge and rub all over the body in a circular motion while showering. A cold shower after cleansing improves the circulation and tightens skin pores.

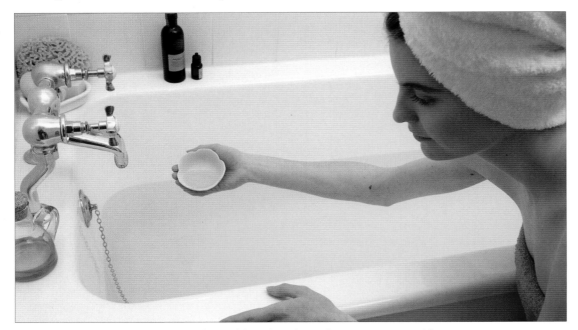

Wait until the bath is almost full before adding the oils, as they evaporate quickly.

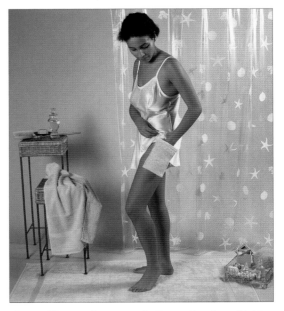

Start off your shower or bath routine by whisking off dead skin cells with a friction mitt. Moisten it with warm water or softening oils such as sweet almond or evening primrose. Concentrate on outer thighs, working from the knee in upward circular movements across the buttocks.

AFTER-BATH BODY TREATMENTS

Moisturizing oils and lotions applied after the bath or shower help to nourish the skin, keeping it soft and supple.
As you get older your skin dehydrates since the oil glands do not produce as much oil as in youth. Apply a body oil all over,
starting from the feet and working right up to the neck and tips of the ears. Avoid talcum powders which clog the pores
and tend to have a drying effect.

PROBLEM ZONES

Pay special attention to your hands, feet and elbows and spend some time each week looking after them.

Hands and nails

Hands and nails take some rough treatment with everyday chores. The ideal time for a manicure or pedicure is after soaking in a bath, when nails and skin have been softened by the water, making it easy to clean around the nail bed and to clip uneven nails without snagging.

Fragile or flaky nails benefit from a rich, nourishing treatment: rub them with apricot kernel, wheat germ or jojoba oil.

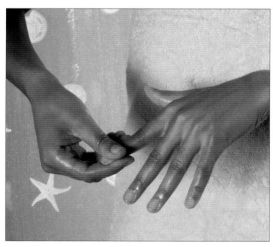

Condition hands and nails with a simple finger-pulling exercise. Spread and stretch the fingers straight out; massage each finger with oil, working from the tip of the nails to the cuticles and up to each knuckle.

RECOMMENDED ESSENTIAL OILS

To soothe and moisturize your hands:
Blend 5 drops each patchouli, lavender and lemon essential oils with 15 ml/1 tbsp sweet almond oil.

For a deodorizing and soothing footbath:
Blend 3 drops each cypress and lavender in a bowl of warm water.

For chilblains:
Blend 3 drops geranium and 1 drop each lavender and rosemary in 15 ml/1 tbsp sweet almond oil.

Body oil formula:
For a lasting effect, mix up to three essential oils, 5 drops of each in 30 ml/2 tbsp base oil. If you want to make up a larger quantity of body oil, use a concentration of 3% essential oil in the base oil.

Feet

Feet are often neglected until they hurt. Polish hard skin with a handful of damp salt or use a pumice stone. While in the bath, bend one knee, grip the toes and then work with the fingers, massaging in an upward direction from the toes to the heels and up the calves in order to stimulate blood flow and relax tired feet. Massage a body oil into the feet after a bath, shower or pedicure.

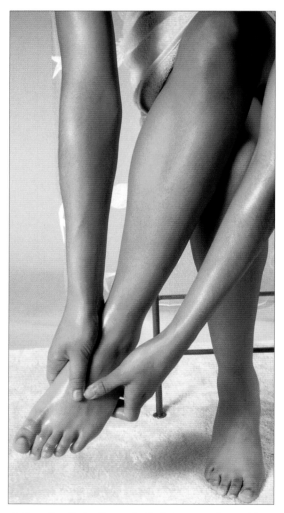

Soften the feet after a bath by massaging with a body oil to which you have added essential oils. Work between the toes and then around the tougher skin and heel areas. Finish with sweeping movements all over to stimulate the circulation.

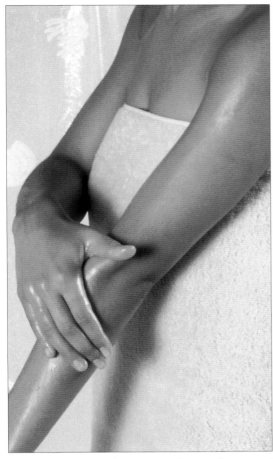

Apply body oil to the arms with smooth upward strokes, concentrating on the elbows and upper arms where the skin is often rougher and drier.

Elbows

Elbows can soon build up hard protective layers of grey, unsightly skin. A good softener for tough elbows is a sweet almond oil and oatmeal scrub. Mix 45 ml/3 tbsp sweet almond oil with 45 ml/3 tbsp fine oatmeal and mix to a paste with fresh milk or yogurt. Smooth and rub over the elbows and any grey, goosey areas of skin around the upper arms. Add 6 drops of fennel essential oil if arms are flabby.

Another great booster for rough elbows is the traditional remedy of cutting a lemon in half, squeezing out the juice and rubbing the elbows in the hollow of the lemon.

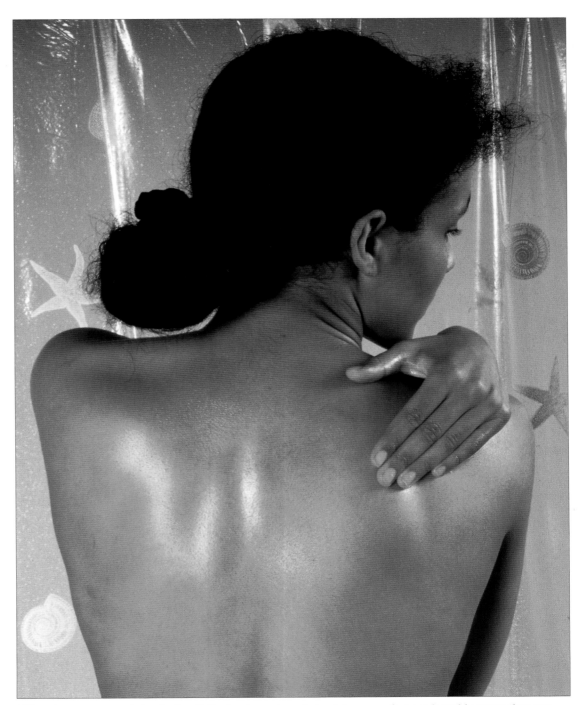

When it comes to applying body oil, the back, neck and shoulders are often neglected because they are difficult to reach, but these are key areas for releasing tension and the skin needs to be nourished, so smooth as far as possible, or enlist the help of a friend.

BEAUTY BASICS

Looking good starts with great skin, and aromatherapy can help you achieve this in various ways: the remarkable penetrative properties of essential oils make them excellent moisturizers, and the wide range of their properties means there is always the right oil for any condition. For instance, rosemary stimulates the circulation and thyme helps the cells to regenerate. As well as being stimulating to the lymphatic system, which helps cleanse the tissue that causes sluggish skin, essential oils can be used as part of your daily skincare routine and to treat specific problems such as acne.

FEED YOUR SKIN

Skin needs to be fed and nourished – inside and out. Healthy diets can keep the body in shape but to keep skin in peak condition it needs to have a ready supply of valuable vitamins and minerals. Many factors can drain the body of this valuable resource – too much over-processed food, caffeine, alcohol, nicotine, sunlight, central heating, carbon monoxide and habitual drug-taking. The effects of these can build up and attack the skin, so from time to time you need to give it a break.

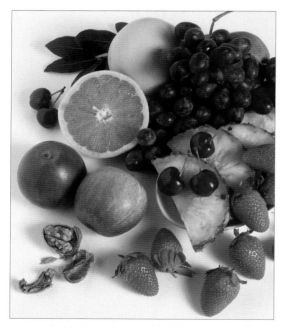

A one-day fruit and vegetable diet is an excellent regime to adopt once a month to cleanse your body and give a boost to your system.

RECOMMENDED ESSENTIAL OILS

For dry skin:
Chamomile, geranium, lavender, hyssop, rose, patchouli, sandalwood, ylang ylang.

For sensitive skin:
Chamomile, lavender, neroli, rose, sandalwood.

For oily skin:
Bergamot, cedarwood, cypress, fennel, lavender, lemon, geranium, juniper, frankincense, sage.

Blends for a facial steam:
Add 5 drops chamomile to a large bowl of hot water for a soothing steam or try lavender, peppermint, thyme or rosemary to stimulate, or comfrey or fennel for their healing properties. Put a towel over your head and lower your face over the steam for 5 minutes.

Nourishing blends for any skin type:
To a 25 g/1 oz pot of unperfumed skin cream, add either 3 drops rose and 3 drops sandalwood, or 4 drops neroli and 2 drops rose.

THE EFFECTS OF STRESS

If you become stressed, the small muscles close to the skin tend to contract. This can leave your skin under-nourished with blood, and over time your complexion and skin tone suffer. Apart from dealing with underlying worries, the skin itself can also be helped with essential oils.

SKIN TYPES

Choose the right oils for your skin type and use them to blend your own cleansers, toners, masks and moisturizers. Remember that skin types can vary: skin may be drier in winter or more prone to oiliness around the time of your period, and it can change as you get older. So review the oils you use to suit your skin now and vary them to meet the changing needs of your complexion.

Combination skin has an oily T-zone from the forehead down to the nose and chin area, and may be normal or dry elsewhere. If you have a complexion like this, double up on the treatments, using oils for oily skin on the greasy patches.

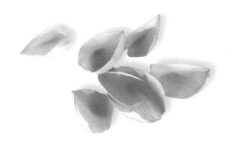

CLEANSERS

Choose the correct essential oils for your skin type and blend them with an ordinary unperfumed brand of cleanser, liquid soap or tissue-off lotion or cream, and they will do nature's work of rebalancing the skin.

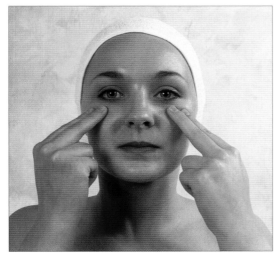

Pay particular attention to oily areas of the face when cleansing the skin.

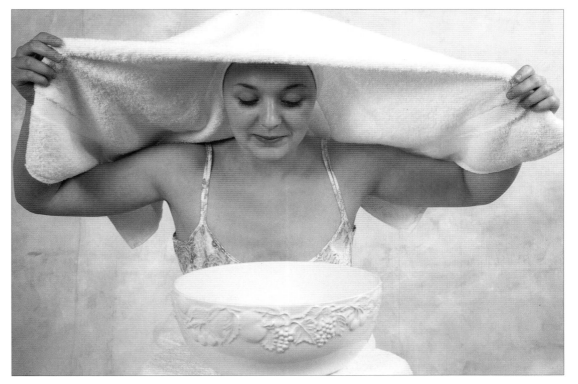

For a deep-cleansing facial steam, boil some water, cool slightly and add 5 drops of essential oil. Put a towel over your head and steam your face for 5 minutes.

TONERS

Essential oils are the gentlest way of toning up. Rose-water for normal or dry/sensitive skin, or witch-hazel for oilier skin, are ideal toners. Or you can blend your own flower waters: simply take a sterile, 100 ml/3½ fl oz bottle of dark-coloured glass, fill it with spring water and add 30 drops of your chosen essential oils. Leave in a cool, dark place for a few days, then filter the water through a coffee filter-paper into a second, similar bottle. Keep it in the fridge.

Herbal infusions also make ideal toners. Boil a cup of water and infuse chamomile, marigold, rosehip or nettle teas. Add 2 drops of orange or lavender oil to the infusion and leave to cool. Oily skin benefits from juniper or lemongrass essential oils, whereas drier skins would appreciate rose or sandalwood.

FACIAL OILS AND CREAMS

Well-moisturized skin is soft and supple, reflects a healthy glow and ages less quickly. Younger skin needs only light conditioning, whereas older skin needs specific nourishing treatments. Most moisturizers soothe and sit on the surface of the skin, but essential oils, with their fine molecular structure, work their way through from the surface to the inner dermis (the skin's deeper regenerating layer). Mixed with the correct amount of base oil, pure essential oils do not clog up the pores: they are light enough to be absorbed spontaneously by the skin.

Use 30 ml/2 tbsp base oil and add 6 drops of essential oils (use a maximum of three different oils) to suit your skin's individual needs. Alternatively, add 6 drops of essential oils to a 25 g/ 1 oz pot of your favourite skin cream.

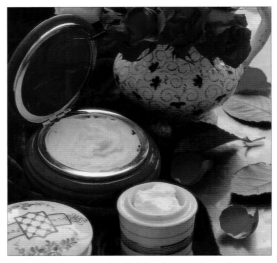

As with all essential oils blends, it is best if you mix up only small amounts of cream and oil at a time to avoid deterioration.

FACE MASKS

Both clay and oatmeal are ideal ingredients for a face mask. Fuller's earth is a natural powdered clay which can be mixed into a paste with hot water. Cool and then add yogurt for a smoother consistency. Similarly, finely ground oatmeal can be mixed into a paste and left to cool. Add 2 drops of essential oils to suit your skin type per 5 ml/1 tsp of paste. Smooth on to your face, leave to dry slightly and then sponge off. For particularly dry sensitive skin, add 5 ml/1 tbsp evening primrose oil to give a more moisturizing mask. When applying, avoid the eye area.

Eye treats

While relaxing with a face mask on, close the eyes and cover them with cotton pads soaked in rosewater, or soothe with two slices of cucumber.

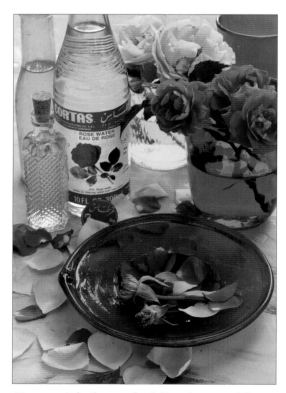

Use essential oils to make delicately-scented flower waters to tone your skin.

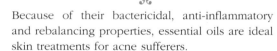

RECOMMENDED ESSENTIAL OILS

A remedy for odd spots:
If you are prone to occasional spots, mix 1 drop of neroli, lemon and lavender in 5 ml/1 tsp base oil and treat just the affected area. For a single spot, use a cotton bud and dab on one spot of undiluted sandalwood.

ACNE

Because of their bactericidal, anti-inflammatory and rebalancing properties, essential oils are ideal skin treatments for acne sufferers.

It is a mistake to scrub oily skin over-zealously: this only activates the sebaceous glands which in turn produce more sebum. If you suffer from pustular acne, avoid excessive facial steams which may spread the condition to other areas of the face: use a mask instead.

From day to day, use a cleanser and moisturizer formulation suitable for sensitive skin, adding 2 drops of juniper, which is stimulating and antiseptic. Opt for a deeper clay-type mask treatment once a week, adding 2 drops of juniper to heal, soothe and tighten the skin, or eucalyptus which is anti-inflammatory, antiseptic and antibiotic. Increase your dietary intake of vitamin E, which is a great skin healer.

COLD SORES

Cold sores are small blisters on the lips or surrounding area which are caused by the virus *Herpes simplex*. It normally lies dormant in nerve cells but can surface when resistance is lowered, such as following a simple cold or 'flu. Any lip sore that persists should be treated medically, but for the common cold sore a dab of undiluted tea tree oil will help.

BROKEN VEINS

These small, red, spider-like thread veins often appear on the surface of the skin around the cheek area. They are broken capillaries and seem to affect those with a delicate or fragile skin type. Hot and cold elements, along with stimulants such as alcohol or caffeine, can trigger this condition. To treat it at home the secret is to protect the skin from losing excess moisture and to give it extra essential oil treatments using parsley, geranium, chamomile, rosemary or cypress in a heavy base oil.

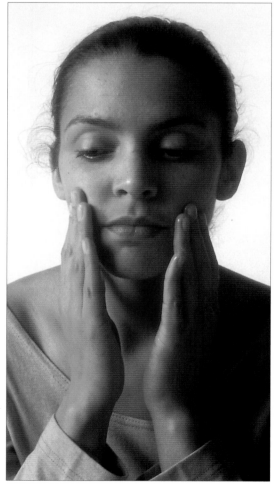

Perfume your favourite face cream with essential oils appropriate to your skin type.

FACIAL MASSAGE

Giving your face a regular massage helps the skin to absorb oils and creams more easily. Give skin a clear start with our step-by-step facial, using a blend of essential oils suited to your skin type in a nourishing carrier oil. This simple routine will tone your skin, helping it to retain its youthful elasticity and smoothing out any fine lines. It will also improve your circulation, speeding up the elimination of toxins from the tissues and giving your face a healthy glow.

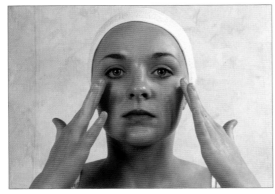

1 Pour a little oil into your hand and apply all over the face, avoiding the eyes.

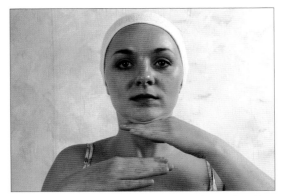

2 With the backs of your hands, gently tap the skin around the jaw line and underneath the chin.

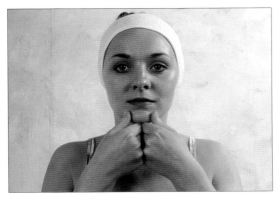

3 Apply small circular movements to the chin area, using your thumbs, to tone, help circulation and eliminate toxins.

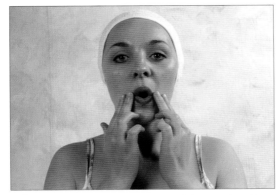

4 Make an "oooh"-shape mouth. Massage the skin on either side of your mouth with your fingertips, easing out fine lines.

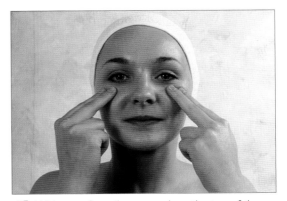

5 With your fingertips, press along the top of the cheekbones and massage outward up to the temples to release toxins.

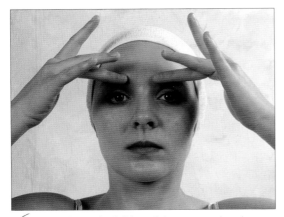

6 Press above the bridge of the nose and under the eyebrows. Hold for 5 seconds, then smooth across the eyebrows and up to the temples.

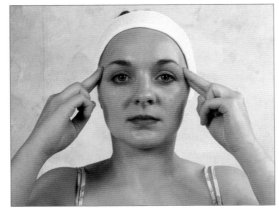

7 To relieve tension, apply firm pressure with the fingertips at either side of the temples and rotate backward.

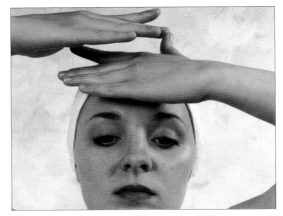

8 Finally, stroke up the forehead from the brow to the hairline with the palm of the hands, smoothing out fine lines.

HEALTHY HAIR

Hair can define your image and style but it is also a mirror of your health. Emotional or physical problems can soon result in a lack of bounce and shine. As with your skin, keeping hair in peak condition is a combination of caring for it on the surface and nurturing it from inside with a well-balanced diet.

HAIR TYPES

How you treat your hair depends largely on its type. Make sure you use the most appropriate treatment for your kind of hair.

Dry hair

Dry hair is rough to touch, thick in texture and dries out at the first sign of heated rollers or tongs. Avoid chemical colorants and perms and opt for shampoos and conditioners containing jojoba and almond oils. Hot-oil treatments allow essential oils to soak in easily and condition the hair. After massaging warm oil into the scalp, wrap the head in a warm towel and leave on for half an hour.

Normal hair

Normal hair is glossy with plenty of natural body and bounce. An occasional hot-oil scalp treatment will keep it looking good and growing healthily.

Greasy hair

Greasy hair tends to look dull, lank, lacks body and won't hold a style. Central heating and environmental elements aggravate the condition, but it can stem from a hormonal imbalance. Check your diet and avoid harsh degreasing shampoos. Clean brushes and combs weekly. Plastic brushes are better for brushing through as bristle continually stimulates the scalp. Choose light conditioning rinses to detangle but try a scalp massage to regulate the oil-producing sebaceous glands.

Combination hair

If the ends of your hair are dry or normal but it is greasy at the roots, avoid using hot appliances near the scalp and keep the ends regularly trimmed. Use a scalp treatment with oils for greasy hair but don't comb through to the ends.

RECOMMENDED ESSENTIAL OILS

For dry hair:
Rose, sandalwood, ylang ylang, lavender, geranium.

For normal hair:
Geranium, lavender, lemongrass, rosemary.

For greasy hair:
Basil, eucalyptus, cedarwood, chamomile, lemongrass, cypress, sage, rosemary.

Scalp massage oil formula:
For the base oil, choose from sweet almond, apricot kernel, avocado, jojoba, evening primrose or sunflower.
Choose up to three essential oils and use 5 drops of each in 30 ml/2 tbsp base oil. Warm the oils by placing the container in a bowl of boiling water, then massage into the scalp. Wrap with a hot towel, leave for 15 minutes and then shampoo.

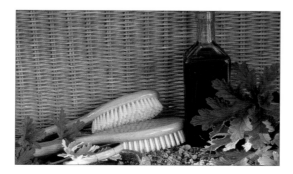

HAIR PROBLEMS

Apart from improving the condition of your hair generally, essential oils can help with specific scalp problems.

Dandruff

There are two types: dry and the more common oily. It's not catching! It can be caused by factors such as chemical body changes, stress, poor eating habits or incorrect application of hair products. Both flaky and dry scalps can be treated with essential oils. Use special dandruff shampoos and conditioning rinses and treat the scalp by gently massaging with suitable oils. For a flaky scalp use patchouli and tea tree. For a dry, itchy scalp, try cedarwood and lavender.

Grey hair

Grey hair is more porous and needs extra conditioning, particularly if it is chemically treated or coloured. Use a blend suitable for dry hair, adding essential oil enhancers like chamomile to lighten or sage to darken any discoloration.

Hair loss

Hair coming out in handfuls is often due to a hormonal imbalance, stress or anxiety, so the first step is to learn to relax. Any unusual thinning patch should be looked at by a trichologist but, as a general remedy, massage the scalp using a blend containing lavender and rosemary oils.

A few drops of geranium oil on a hairbrush add a delightful fragrance to the hair, while chamomile makes an excellent rinse for fair hair.

SCALP MASSAGE

This is a wonderful way to condition hair, stimulate the scalp and relieve tension. You can use these steps to treat your own hair, but it's even more relaxing if you can persuade a friend to help, especially if your hair is long.

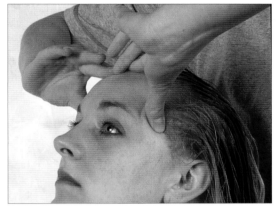

1 Shampoo the hair and towel dry. Comb through with a wide-tooth comb. Tilt your head back and pour some blended oil on to the hairline, massaging in with thumbs on the temples and fingers spread apart over the centre of the head.

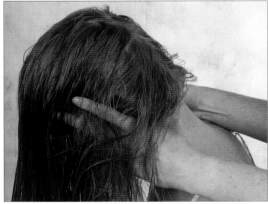

4 Work from front to back, following the natural flow of blood, from the forehead, frontal hairline, temples and sides, over the crown of the head to the base of the neck. If the scalp feels particularly tight, concentrate on areas where it doesn't want to move. At the base of the skull, press firmly and push the whole scalp up toward the crown to release tension.

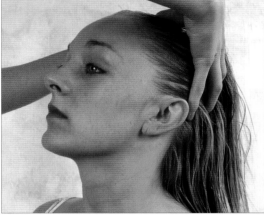

2 Loosely run fingers and oil over the top of the scalp from front to back, lifting hair at the crown. Keep dipping your fingertips in the oil as you begin the massage so that there is enough on the hair to spread right through to the ends.

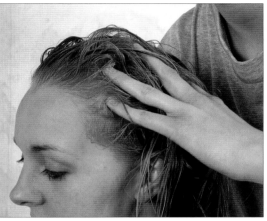

3 Massage the head with kneading movements. Grip and push against the scalp, which should gently rotate against the skull. Concentrate on one area at a time, with the hands positioned on either side of the scalp.

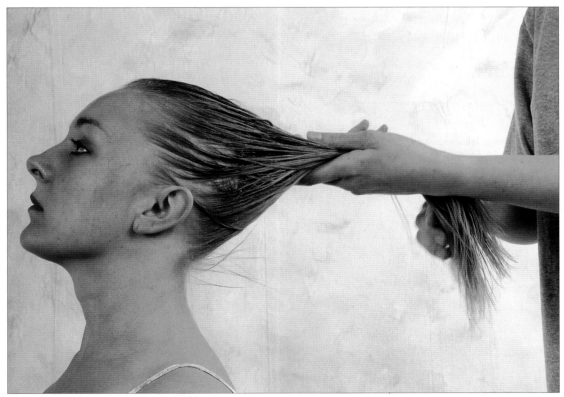

5 Pull any extra oil through the hair, working out from the roots to the ends. Make sure all the hair is well oiled, then wrap it in a towel and leave for at least 15 minutes before shampooing.

AROMATHERAPY MASSAGE

An aromatherapy massage is a wonderful way to unwind and ease stored tensions, triggering the body's natural healing processes by stimulating the flow of blood and lymph fluid. At the same time, the aromas are acting upon the emotional centre in the brain (the limbic system) which governs the way you feel.

CHOOSING ESSENTIAL OILS FOR MASSAGE

Aromatherapists never start a massage immediately. In order to provide the most effective treatment, the therapist needs to ascertain the state of mind and body of the individual, and establish whether there are any specific problems to attend to. Is the problem physical? Is it mental? Is it a combination of both? To help them to treat a wide variety of complaints, aromatherapists have many oils at their fingertips, but they never mix or use them until they have worked out a prescription for the receiver's individual needs.

Mixing oils is a skilled art, but there are simple recipes, such as those suggested throughout this book, that you can use at home to deal with specific problems from muscular aches and pains to headaches and stress. With potent essential oils it is far better to use less, rather than more, so if in doubt start the massage with a carrier oil such as sweet almond to which you have added 2–3 drops of just one essential oil. Lavender, rosemary and geranium are good, all-purpose oils, or you could use chamomile for particularly sensitive skin.

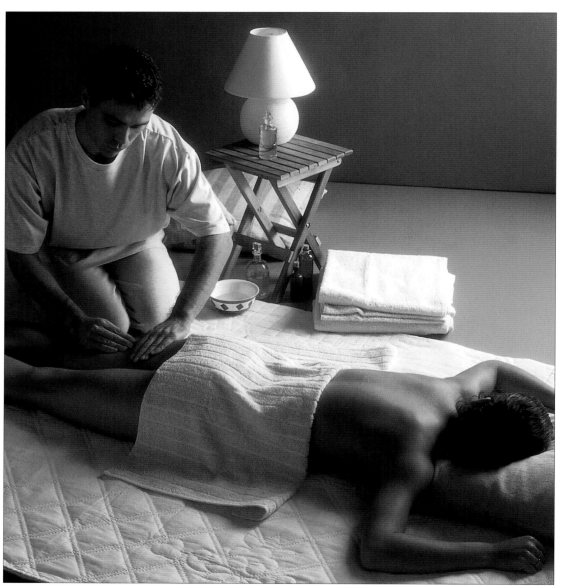

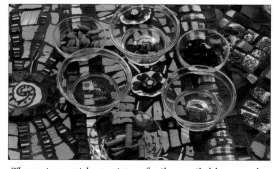

There is a wide variety of oils available – make sure you choose the right one for your partner.

Create a warm, relaxing environment with soft lighting and a comfortable base for your partner to lie on. Play gentle music in the background, and warm the towels before you begin.

GIVING THE MASSAGE

- Before you give a massage to a partner, try out the movements on parts of your own body to get a sense of how the strokes should feel and how much pressure to use.
- Always warm your hands before you begin to apply the oil.
- If the part of the body you're working on is particularly hairy or the skin is very dry, you will need to apply more oil.
- Massage movements should be slow and gentle to help relaxation and eliminate tension which tightens the muscles.
- Remember that the movements should flow into each other. If you find that you have missed out a step or gone on to the wrong part of the body, don't panic. Finish the part you are working on before going back to it, or leave it out altogether rather than interrupting the flow of the massage.
- When you give the massage, make sure you are relaxed and comfortable, as well as your partner, or you will transmit your own tensions and it will not be an effective massage.
- Try to maintain contact with your partner's body as much as possible; even as you move into a different position, try to keep a hand on their body.
- Keep your touch light and sensitive. Remember that your hands are the main channel of communication during the massage.

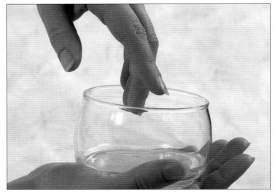

Keep the oil in an easy dispenser or bowl so you don't have to worry about lids during the massage. But keep the oil covered in some way, as essential oils will quickly evaporate.

RECEIVING THE MASSAGE

Bear the following points in mind when you are planning to have an aromatherapy massage so that you get the most benefit from the treatment.

Before the massage

- Have a cool shower or wash: don't soak in a hot bath, or the oils will immediately seep into the skin.
- Don't use an underarm deodorant or body spray before the treatment, as this will block the effect of the oils.
- Don't have a large meal just before an aromatherapy massage as the body's systems will have to work too hard at digesting to be thoroughly relaxed.
- Don't drink alcohol before a treatment.

- Don't have a massage if you have 'flu or a fever or any serious condition. Wait until you are over the worst, then let an aromatherapy treatment help restore your system's balance.

After the massage

- Lie still for at least 5 minutes before getting up at the end of the treatment.
- Drink a glass of still water immediately after a treatment.
- Don't bathe or shower for at least 12 hours after a treatment to allow the oils to be absorbed by the skin and begin the all-important work of detoxifying the body.
- Drink plenty of water for the rest of the day as the kidneys will be active in eliminating toxins.
- Avoid alcohol for at least 12 hours after the treatment to give the body a chance to detoxify.

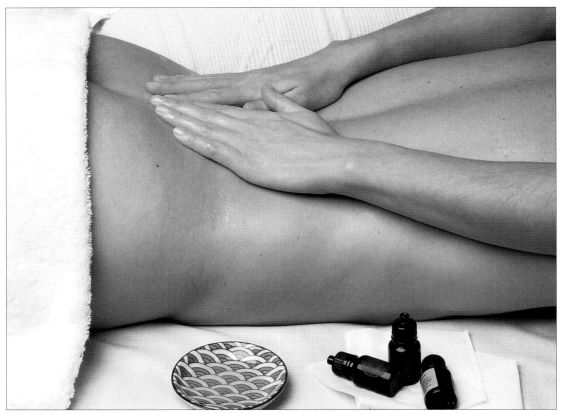

Begin the massage with long, calm, flowing strokes to relax your partner both physically and psychologically.

PREPARATION AND EQUIPMENT FOR MASSAGE

A successful massage benefits and relaxes both body and mind, and careful preparation prior to the session helps to achieve this aim. This involves creating a natural and nurturing ambience, as well as having everything you need to hand. Your preparation will give you confidence and trust in your abilities, and your partner will instinctively feel safe in your hands, knowing that you value and respect their comfort and needs. In an atmosphere of mutual relaxation, your massage can proceed in a calm and serene manner.

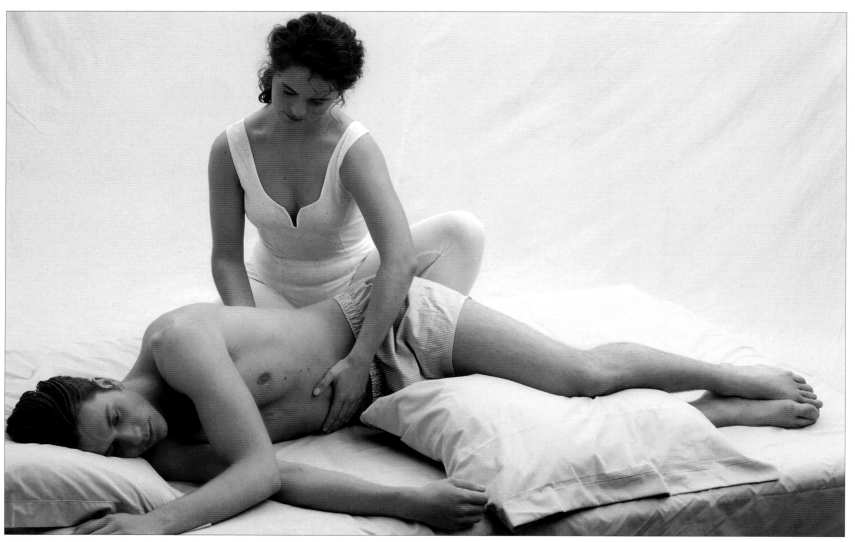

A futon is ideal for massage, but a foam rubber mattress placed on the floor is a suitable alternative. Wear clean, light, comfortable clothing that is not too tight when giving a massage. Remember that giving a massage is quite energetic and you will get warmer as you proceed.

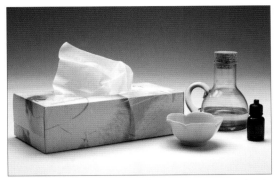

Have all materials and equipment ready in advance of the massage, including tissues and oils.

THE SETTING

Most rooms can be easily converted into a peaceful setting. Soft, diffused lighting will enhance a tranquil mood. Ensure that the room you choose is warm and draught-free, as body temperature is likely to drop rapidly while lying still, especially when your partner is covered in oil. As the giver of the massage, be aware of the discrepancy between your body temperature and that of your partner. Wear light, comfortable clothing while giving the massage.

Privacy and quiet is essential to relaxation during massage. Pick a time when you will not be disturbed or hurried, bearing in mind that a complete massage may last between an hour and an hour-and-a-half.

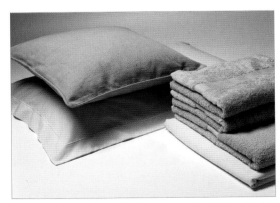

All sheets, towels and pillowcases should be freshly laundered for each session.

EQUIPMENT

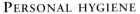

Have a pile of fresh, clean towels and sheets ready for use. Cover the surface your partner will be lying on with a sheet. Have several pillows or thinly folded towels ready to place beneath the body to ease areas of tension. If the massage will take place at floor level, use cushions to kneel or sit on for your own comfort.

The massage base must be firm, comfortable and supportive. A futon or foam rubber mattress is ideal, or you can provide adequate padding with folded blankets. Beds are generally too soft unless you are stroking only very lightly. Ensure that the area surrounding the massage base is uncluttered so you have maximum freedom of movement.

Have all your aromatherapy materials and equipment ready for use before the session begins. Under some circumstances it may be preferable to use the selected essential oils in a vaporizer rather than blend them with the massage oil. Tissues or small towels should be available for wiping oil from your hands, or for your partner's convenience. If you are concerned about oil stains, place a thin rubber sheet under the massage sheet, or a beautician's tissue couch roll or a bath towel over the top of the sheet. If essential oil is accidentally spilt on clothing, dab it off quickly with a tissue. It will soon evaporate but it may leave a stain, so rinse out clothing in warm soapy water.

PERSONAL HYGIENE

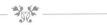

This is very important for both participants. Make certain you come to the session freshly showered, with clean nails, hands and feet. Wipe your hands after massaging the feet before proceeding with strokes on other parts of the body. Always wash your hands thoroughly at the end of each massage session.

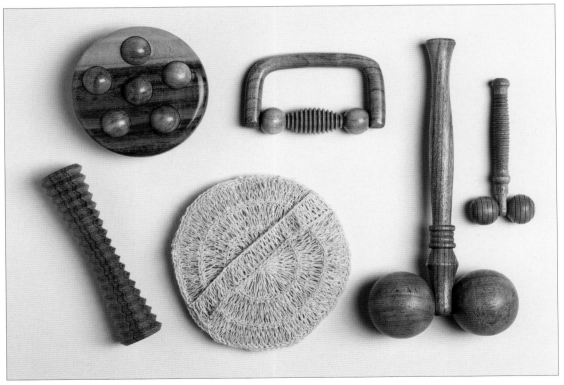

Wooden massage tools in various shapes are particularly useful for self-massage.

THE BASIC TECHNIQUES OF MASSAGE

The following pages introduce the basic techniques of massage, which will help you build up a flowing sequence of strokes and enable you to bring a harmonious state of relaxation and invigoration to your partner.

KEEPING YOUR PARTNER COMFORTABLE

Use warmed, fresh, clean towels to cover your partner during massage. The towels will prevent the loss of body heat once the oil has been applied and the person is lying still. They also ensure your partner's modesty is respected. Move the towels as needed while applying your strokes, leaving uncovered only the area on which you are working during the massage.

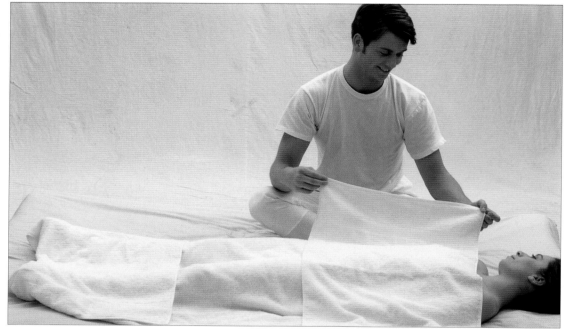

1 Ideally you should use one large bath towel to cover the whole body, and two medium-sized towels to add further warmth to the upper body and the feet. Tuck the towel snugly around both feet.

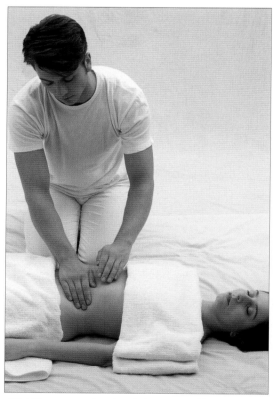

2 When massaging the abdomen, peel back the large towel and cover the breasts with a folded towel. Do not leave the chest and breasts exposed.

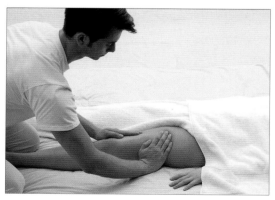

3 Once you are working on the legs, ensure that the upper body stays warm by covering it with an extra towel. Fold the large towel over so that only the leg on which you are working remains exposed.

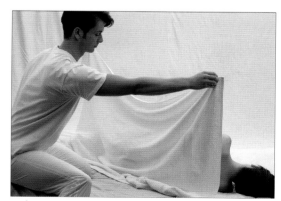

4 When your partner turns over, hold the towel up between you both, and then let it drop softly down on the other side of the body.

BEGINNING THE MASSAGE

After you have decided on the blend of essential oils you will be using for the massage, give your partner time to undress and make themselves comfortable and relaxed while you mix the oils. Take a few moments to calm yourself and centre your thoughts before you begin. Your first contact with your partner should be steady and reassuring.

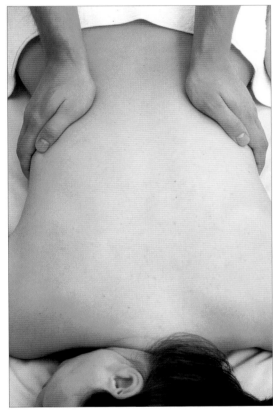

1 Rub a little of your chosen blend of oil into the palms of your hands and spread it over the area you intend to massage with the flat of the hands, in smooth, flowing motions. For the initial stroke, the flowing motion should define the contours of the whole of the area you intend to massage. While integrating the whole surface of the body, this stroke also warms the muscles and prepares them for subsequent massage techniques. The integration stroke is usually a large, flowing and continuous motion, which is repeated 3–5 times for full effect.

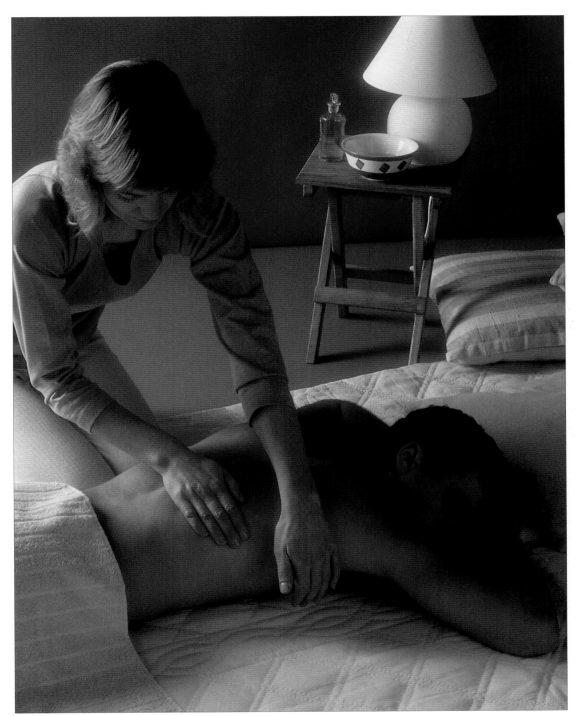

Arrange the mattress or futon on which your partner is to lie so that there is sufficient space for you to move freely around it.

EFFLEURAGE

Effleurage is the first and main stroke of massage. It prepares the body's soft tissues and warms the muscles for all deeper movements. It is also used to follow up more vigorous strokes such as kneading and friction, in order to soothe and relax an area that has just been massaged. Effleurage simply means "stroking", and is a free-flowing, continuous movement made with the flat of one or, more usually, both hands at a steady pressure.

Effleurage strokes have a calming and almost hypnotic effect on the body, allowing a sense of trust to develop so that the recipient can relax both physically and psychologically. The strokes can be applied with a light to medium pressure, with the whole hand in contact with the skin. When applied in a movement up towards the heart, these strokes benefit the cardiovascular system (the heart and network of blood vessels) and the lymphatic system by boosting the circulation of blood and lymph around the body. A lighter movement has a calming effect on the function of the nervous system.

While making the strokes, the hands should be completely relaxed so that they mould themselves into the body's contours and define its shape. Effleurage has a fluid quality so that the strokes flow around the body and never finish abruptly.

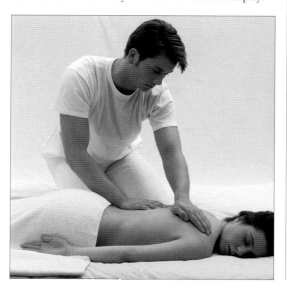

FANNING

Fanning is an effleurage movement that can be applied to many areas of the body, including the back, chest, legs and arms. It is an excellent stroke to follow on from larger preparatory movements and can be used to stretch and manipulate tension away from the muscles. Fanning can be applied either as a series of shorter movements for remedial effect or in larger, more flowing motions for sensual and soothing effects. Use a steady pressure for the upward stroke and keep the movement slow and relaxed.

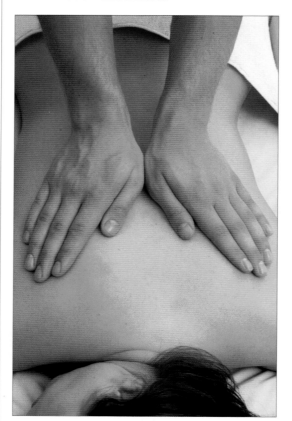

1 Place both hands flat on either side of the spine with the fingers together, pointing straight up towards the head. Keeping the whole hand in contact with the skin, stroke with an even pressure for about 15 cm/6 in up the back. Now let your hands flow outwards in a fanning motion, moving away from each other towards the sides of the ribcage.

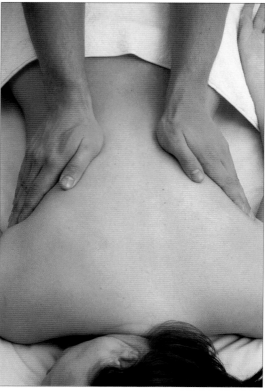

2 Shape your hands to the sides of the body, then draw the hands down before sliding them lightly around and towards their original position alongside the spine. Now stroke further up the back.

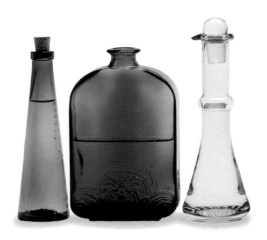

CONTINUOUS CIRCLE STROKES

Continuous circle strokes add a sensual, relaxing and soporific element to the massage. If applied at a more vigorous pace and with slightly firmer pressure, they are excellent for warming the superficial layers of tissue and for releasing tension. These effleurage strokes can be used on any broad expanse of the body, such as the sides of the ribcage, the back and the thighs, when they are applied in a flowing, unbroken motion. Continuous circle strokes also form the main preparatory strokes on the abdomen.

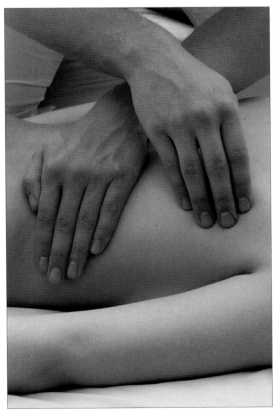

2 While your left hand continues to make a full circle, the right hand lifts up and passes over the top of the moving left hand.

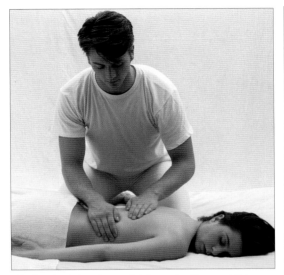

1 Lay both hands parallel to each other and flat on the area you intend to massage. The hands should be both flexible and soft enough to mould into the body's contours. Begin to slide both hands in the same direction in a circular motion.

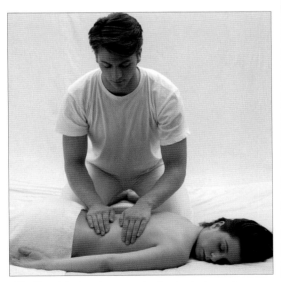

3 The right hand returns to the body to perform a half-circle stroke before lifting off again to let the left hand complete the next full circular motion.

KNEADING

Kneading is one of the most satisfying strokes in massage both to give and to receive, because it takes hold of the muscle and moves it about, creating greater flexibility and suppleness. To knead well, the hands should be dextrous and pliable; the motion is similar to the action of a baker kneading dough.

Kneading is a lifting, squeezing and rolling movement that passes the flesh from one hand to the other. It has a rhythmic, circular motion and should be applied with the wrists and shoulders relaxed, and the arms held at a distance from the body. Stand or kneel on the opposite side of the body, so that your fingers are pointing downwards as you work.

Kneading is a good stroke to apply on muscular and fleshy areas such as the calves, thighs, buttocks and waist after they have been relaxed and warmed by effleurage. It benefits the muscles by releasing underlying tension, breaking down fat deposits and toxins trapped in the tissues and aiding the exchange of tissue fluids. Always follow up kneading with effleurage strokes to soothe the area and boost the blood and lymph circulation so that released toxins can be properly eliminated from the body.

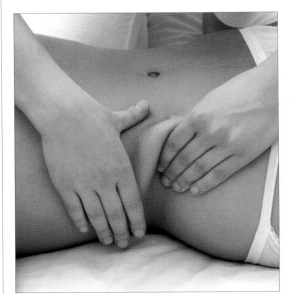

FRICTION AND PRESSURE STROKES

Friction and pressure strokes work on releasing tension by pushing the muscle down towards the bone and then stretching it. Apply after kneading on fleshy areas, or following effleurage wherever the bone is close to the surface of the skin, such as on the hands, feet, face or alongside the spine. A pressure stroke is made by leaning your weight steadily into muscle or connective tissue. The heel of the hand, thumb pads, finger pads, knuckles and forearm can all be used. The pressure must always be applied and released slowly and sensitively.

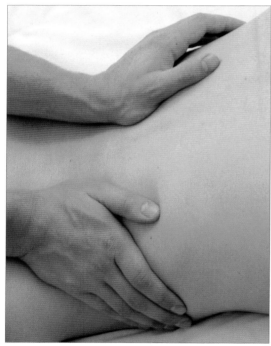

1 The heel of the hand provides a broad, flat surface with which to add pressure during massage, and it is particularly effective in stretching and draining muscle in tight areas such as the lower back and thighs. Shift the weight in the hands into the heels and use in alternating, circular motions – one hand following the other in a continuous flow of movement. The pressure should be applied in the upward and outward half of the slide, but decreased in the last half of the circle as the hands glide softly around to repeat the stroke.

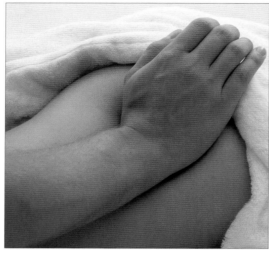

2 By keeping the whole hand relaxed but applying direct pressure into the heel, these circular motions will ease tension from the muscles of the buttocks.

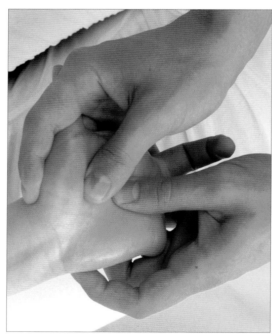

4 Support the back of your partner's hand with your fingers and use small and continuously alternating thumb circles over the palms and wrists to remove stiffness. To achieve the correct movement in these strokes, you must rotate the thumbs from their base joint.

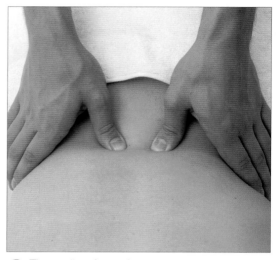

3 The small surfaces of the thumb pads are able to penetrate into those areas where muscles and tendons are attached to bone, for example alongside the spine. Painful tight spots can be eased by leaning weight into the thumbs while the hands remain relaxed on the body, and then making a good firm sliding motion up each side of the spine.

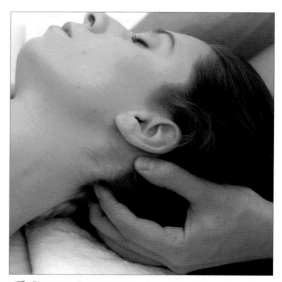

5 Finger pad pressure can be applied to release tension from under bone, such as the ridge of the skull. The pressure must be applied slowly to allow your partner time to relax. Slowly rotate your fingertips on one area at a time. Then release the pressure gradually before moving to the next spot.

PERCUSSION

Percussion strokes include a variety of invigorating movements that briskly strike fleshy and muscular areas of the body to produce a toning and stimulating effect on the skin. They are performed with one hand following the other in a series of rapid and rhythmic movements, helping to draw the blood towards the skin's surface and leaving it with a warm and healthy glow. The rapid action also dispels tension and rids the tissues of excess fluid and fatty deposits. To achieve the best results, keep your shoulders, wrists and hands relaxed, and bounce your hands immediately back off the skin the moment they make contact.

The invigorating effects of percussion help to enliven the body after the euphoric effects of other massage strokes, but they may not be suitable to use if your partner is in a particularly sensitive or vulnerable mood. Percussion strokes should never be applied over varicose veins or directly on top of bone.

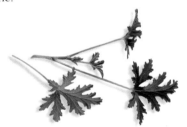

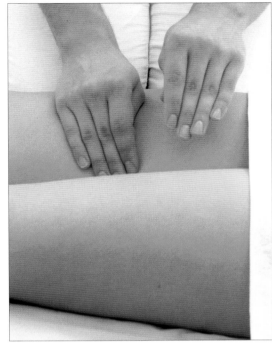

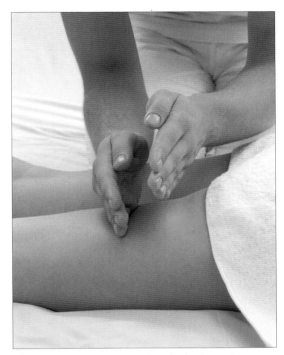

1 To perform the cupping movement, form both hands into a softly cupped shape by keeping your fingers straight but bent at the lower knuckles; at the same time draw the thumbs close into the palms. This should create an airtight vacuum in the centre of your palms, which exerts suction on the skin during the rapid cupping action. Using the palms to make contact, briskly strike and flick off the skin, one hand following the other in quick succession over fleshy areas.

2 Hacking uses the same fast rhythmic motion as cupping, but contact with the skin is made from the sides of the hands, one following the other in quick succession. The wrists and fingers should be relaxed and the palms of each hand should face each other with only about 2.5 cm/1 in between them. Hacking tones and stimulates all fleshy areas, and works particularly well on the buttocks, thighs and tops of the shoulders.

3 For the pummelling stroke, keep your shoulders and wrists relaxed and make loose fists in order to pummel over the fleshy parts of your partner's body. Contact with the skin is made with the sides of the hands. Apply the stroke in the same brisk fashion as the previous percussion strokes, letting one hand after the other pummel over the area you are massaging. This stroke, applied to the thighs and buttocks, is excellent for helping to break down cellulite.

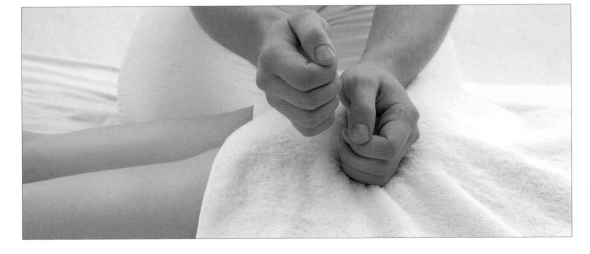

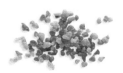

APPLYING THE CORRECT SEQUENCE OF STROKES

The following sequence of strokes on the calf muscles of the leg shows the order in which the basic techniques of massage should be applied to create a relaxing and invigorating effect. This sequence can be used, as appropriate, on any part of the body.

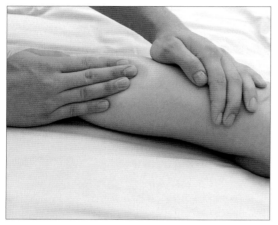

1 *Effleurage*: Soothing strokes made with the flat of the hands will warm and loosen tense calf muscles and prepare them for deeper strokes.

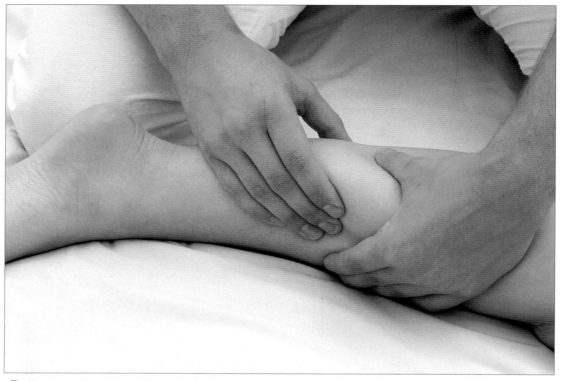

2 *Kneading*: Knead the calf muscles to invigorate the muscles and help them to contract. Follow up with some soft strokes.

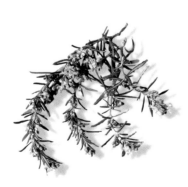

3 *Friction*: Press your thumb pads sensitively into the muscle tissue using alternating thumb circle friction strokes. This will stretch and release a deeper level of tension. Work thoroughly over the whole area.

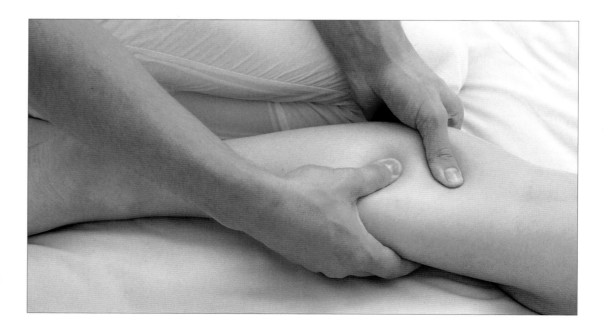

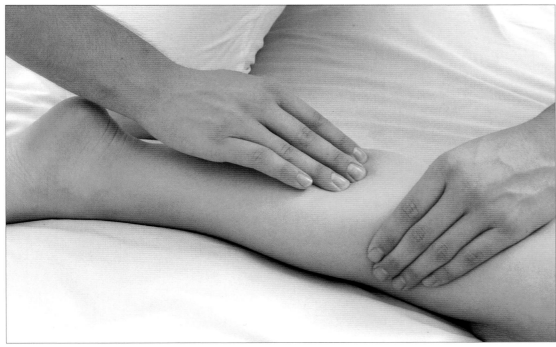

4 *Vibrating*: Gently sink your fingertips into the calf muscle and vibrate it rapidly. Let your hands mould into the shape of the lower leg as you follow the vibrating action with flowing effleurage.

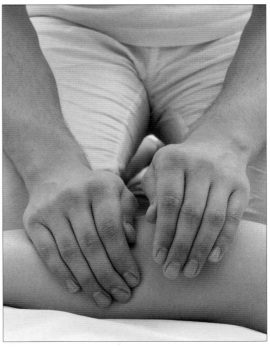

5 *Cupping*: Cup the calf briskly to stimulate the blood circulation and tone the skin and the muscles. Apply the cupping motion up and down the lower leg several times.

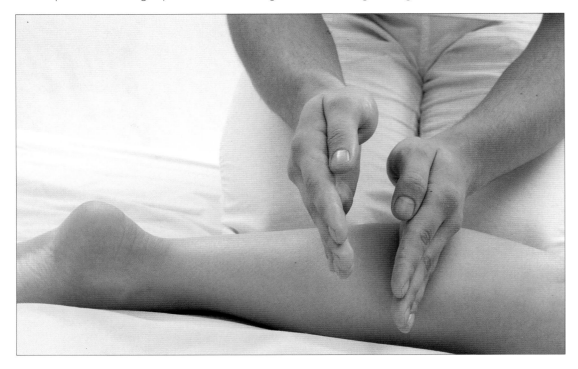

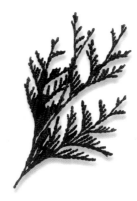

6 *Hacking*: Use the hacking stroke over the bulk of the calf muscles for further toning, and to aid the elimination of excess tissue fluids. Do not strike the back of the knee. *Stroking*: Gently stroke over the calf as in step 1, to harmonize the previous massage movements and to boost both the blood and lymph circulation towards the heart.

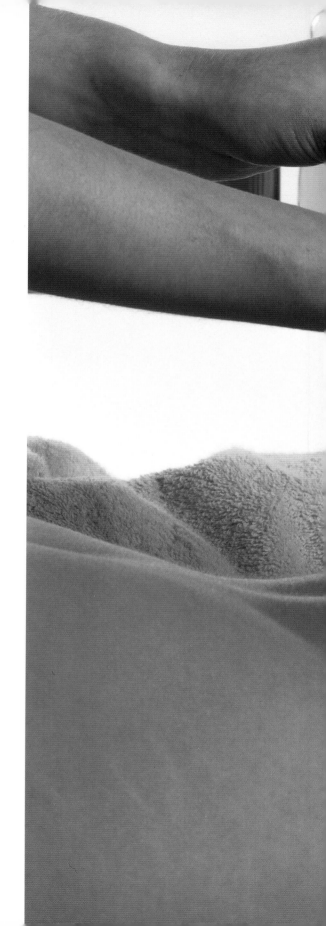

OILS IN THERAPY

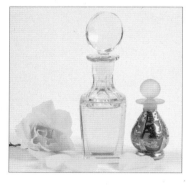

Aromatherapy treats both mind and body, working mainly on the nervous system, and is able both to relax and stimulate. When it is used in massage, the highly potent essential oils penetrate the body via the skin and are also inhaled as the treatment progresses. While the techniques and strokes of massage can ease pain or tension from stiff and aching muscles, boost a sluggish circulation or eliminate toxins, at the same time the nurturing touch of the hands on the body soothes away mental stress and restores emotional equilibrium.

The use of essential oils in therapy can help to alleviate specific symptoms, but can also help to promote a more balanced and healthy lifestyle. There is less likelihood of succumbing to everyday illnesses such as colds, and of suffering from the effects of stress. A balanced state of mind promotes vitality and a better ability to cope with potentially difficult events or situations, such as a crisis at work, an interview, or even a visit to the dentist. The use of aromatherapy can also stimulate the immune system, avoiding the run down feeling which can lead to flu-like symptoms or general weariness. The following pages are a guide to the use of oils in the alleviation of complaints such as headache, nausea and the symptoms of flu, stress and bad circulation.

Massage with essential oils works both physically and
psychologically to relax and stimulate the nervous system.

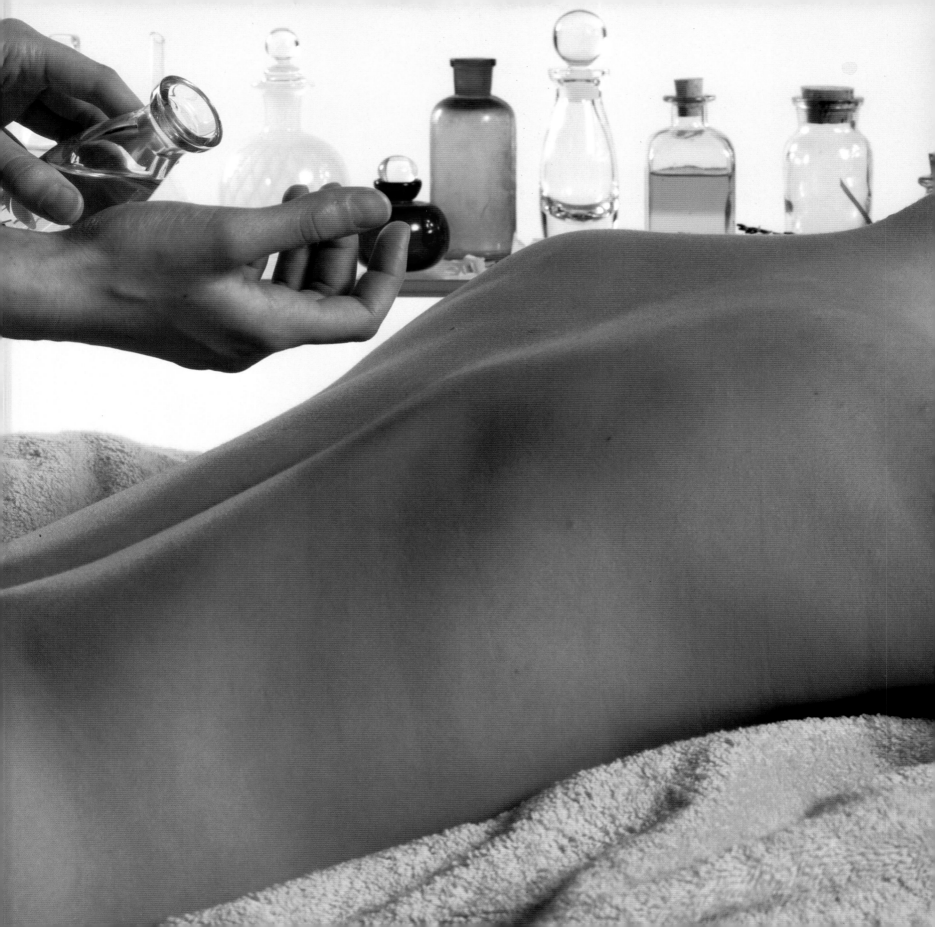

EASING HEADACHES AND MIGRAINES

Most headaches are caused by tension, but occasionally they are the result of an allergic reaction to food or a symptom of an ailment such as sinusitis. Whatever the cause, gentle massage at the earliest moment can help to stop headaches from getting a tight grip. Compresses are another option: a cold compress of lavender or geranium across the forehead will provide pleasant relief, or for tension in the neck sandalwood can be helpful.

RELEASING CONSTRICTED MUSCLES

It is thought that tension headaches are caused by a change in blood pressure brought about when muscles tense and restrict blood flow. The main areas of muscular tension are the shoulders, neck and below the ridge of the skull.

RECOMMENDED ESSENTIAL OILS

To relieve a tension headache or migraine:
Lavender.

If the headache is the result of overwork, anger or worry:
Chamomile or marjoram.
For a sharp, piercing pain;
if the head feels hot:
Peppermint.

For a feeling of lethargy and despondency:
Lemon or rosemary.

To relieve the symptoms of colds
and sinusitis:
Eucalyptus.

At the earliest stages of a migraine,
blend 2 drops rosemary, 1 drop each
marjoram and clary sage.

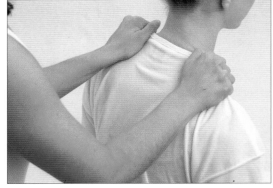

1 Rest one hand on each shoulder for a few moments, then, anchoring your fingers over the top of the shoulders, roll and squeeze the muscles in a kneading action, using the heels of your hands. Work out to the edge of the shoulders and down the tops of the arms.

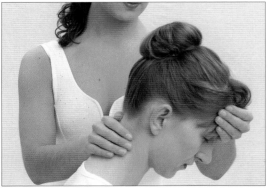

2 Place one hand across the forehead and the other across the nape of the neck. Ask your partner to drop her head into your hand and breathe gently, imagining that she is releasing tension with each out-going breath. Gently squeeze the neck muscles between the fingers and heel of your hand.

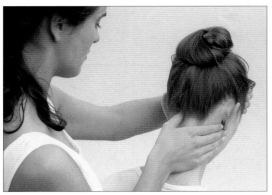

3 Still supporting the forehead, use the thumb pad of the other hand to press upwards into the hollow at the top of the spine. Apply gentle pressure for a steady count of five, then release.

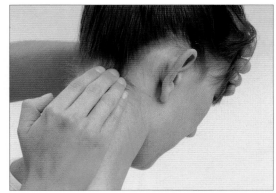

4 Loosen the constricted muscles under the base of the skull by massaging beneath the bony ridge, working from the top of the spine to the outer edge of the skull. Change hands to massage the other side. Ease scalp tension by rotating the fingertips of both hands in small circles all over the head.

STRETCHING THE NECK MUSCLES

Tense neck muscles can be eased through gentle stretching. It is important to make sure your partner is lying perfectly straight before you begin.

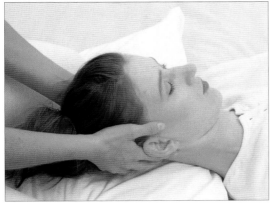

1 Slip both hands under your partner's shoulders, with your fingers resting at the top of the spine and your palms supporting the back of the neck. Ask your partner to relax her neck into your hands, then pull them steadily upwards to stretch and lengthen the neck away from the shoulders. Raise her head slightly as your hands pass under the hairline and up the back of the head.

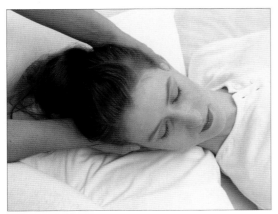

2 Cup the head in your hands, with your fingers resting on the neck and your thumbs lying gently against the sides of the face. Encouraging your partner to relax completely, lift the head slightly, then roll it gently to the right and to the left. Repeat this action several times.

DRAWING OUT THE PAIN

These four techniques all involve applying pressure then releasing it, to relax muscles and lift the pain of a tension headache away from the head.

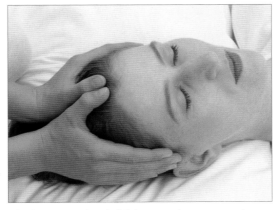

1 Settle your hands lightly around your partner's scalp for a few moments. Keeping your hands in the cupped position, lift them slowly away from the head as if they were drawing out the pain.

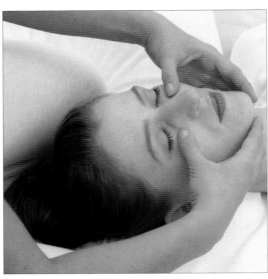

3 Working from inner to outer edge, apply a press/release motion under the ridge of both eyebrows using the tips of your index fingers. Then use your thumb pads to press/release over the top of the cheekbones, working out from the nose to the edge of the temples.

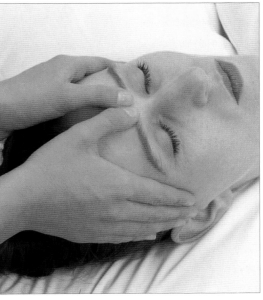

2 Cup your hands around the head again, placing your thumbs between the eyebrows. Apply gentle pressure with your thumbs for a count of five, then release the pressure.

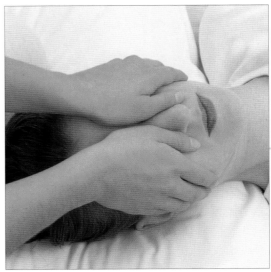

4 Briskly rub your hands together to create heat, then softly lay your slightly cupped palms over the eyes for a count of five to soothe and relax the eye muscles. Withdraw your hands slowly.

CALMING ANXIETY AND STRESS

Aromatherapy and massage provide excellent antidotes to the symptoms of anxiety and stress. A prolonged state of anxiety can deplete vital energy from the body, leading to a general state of nervousness and tension. While essential oils will soothe and comfort, massage strokes will return a sense of physical reality, helping to calm the anxiety.

Anxiety can be alleviated with a combination of uplifting and calming oils, used in an aromatic bath or blended into a massage oil. Whichever oils you choose, use two relaxing oils to one uplifting one.

To prevent undue stress, when you find yourself in a potentially stressful situation try simply inhaling one of your favourite oils at regular intervals. Alternatively, you could put a couple of drops of a relaxing oil such as lavender or geranium in a vaporizer in your room or office to help keep you feeling more relaxed and calm.

RECOMMENDED ESSENTIAL OILS

To aid relaxation and reduce the effects of stress:
Lavender, geranium, marjoram.

To comfort and lift the spirits:
Basil, clary sage, ylang ylang.

If the anxiety attack causes a digestive upset:
Neroli.

To alleviate a sense of alienation:
Sandalwood, rosewood or frankincense.

Blend 5 drops each basil, neroli and lavender with 15 ml/1 tbsp carrier oil to use as a restorative bath oil.

SOOTHING AWAY STRESS

Releasing tension from the brow, temples, jaw and neck will help to calm the mind.

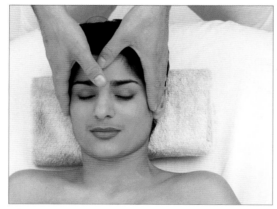

1 Using your thumbs in the centre of the forehead, stroke one after the other in short, firm slides, to ease the tension from the area between, and directly above, the eyebrows.

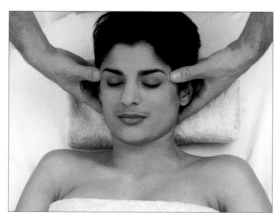

3 Placing your fingers around the back of the head, use the thumbs to stroke in soft, circular motions over the temples.

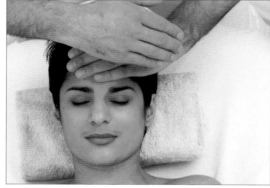

2 Using the palms and fingers, brush your hands soothingly in alternating motions from one side of the forehead to the other. With the fingers of your right hand pointing to the left temple, draw your hand lightly across the brow, before lifting it off to let your left hand repeat the motion from the right temple.

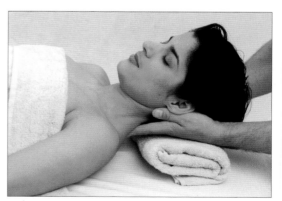

4 Releasing and extending the neck will loosen constricted muscles. Place both hands, fingers pointing downwards, along each side of the top of the spine. Ask your partner to breathe deeply and relax her neck and head back into your hands. Pull your hands gently, with the fingertips slightly indented into the tissue, up the back of the neck and out from under the head.

THE SOLAR PLEXUS STROKE

This is a marvellous way of unlocking tension by calming the main nerves that run through this area in the centre of the body. Use your left hand (for calming) to stroke the solar plexus (located just below the breast bone) in anti-clockwise circles. Close your eyes as you do this and try to empty your mind of the anxious thoughts that are making you feel tense, concentrating instead on what you are doing. This calming action can help soothe you even if you do it through your clothes, but the effect is enhanced if you use a relaxing essential oil on the skin, such as lavender or geranium. Try it while your bath is running, or when lying in bed before you go to sleep.

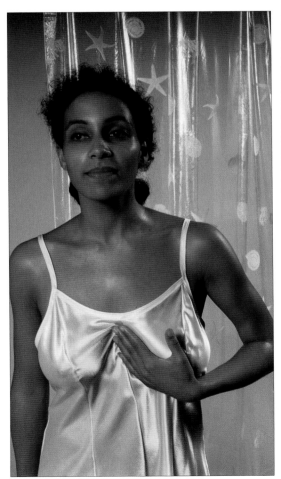

PULSING THE JOINTS

Passive movements to loosen and relax the joints of the body will help to release tension. It is important to encourage your partner to give up the control of movement and weight of her limbs into your hands, thereby enabling her to trust you and free her tension. Gently rotate, wiggle, stretch and rock the joints of the body in line with their natural movement. Encourage your partner to breathe into these areas to allow a greater sense of connection to her body. You can follow up these passive movements with massage on the arms, hands, legs and feet to release tension. Never try to force someone into relaxing, however, and always respect their level of tension.

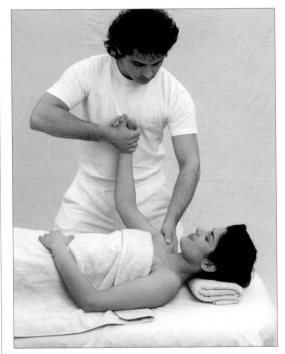

1 Keeping the elbow slightly flexed, lift the arm away from the body. To secure your hold, clasp the wrist and hand and slip your thumb between your partner's thumb and index finger. Place your other hand supportively behind the shoulder. Rock the arm gently so that the movement travels up into the shoulder joint. Lift and lower the arm as you rock it to encourage a complete release of tension.

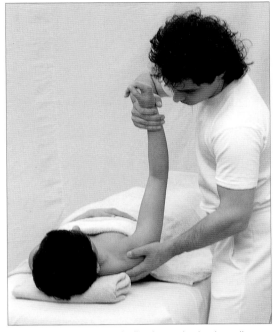

2 Lifting the arm vertically above the body, pull gently upwards to create an easy stretch in the joint before slowly releasing the traction. Then, with the elbow slightly flexed, bounce the arm gently up and down into the shoulder socket, and against the support of your hand.

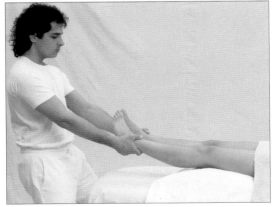

3 A gentle stretch in the legs releases tension from the hips and pelvis. Positioning yourself below your partner's feet, clasp the back of both ankles with your hands. Lean back in your own body to pull her legs towards you, and then slowly and easily release this traction.

INSOMNIA

Sleeplessness is a common response to stress, as your mind and body refuse to let go enough to give you the rest that you need. The resulting disturbed and restless night leaves you more prone to stress and anxiety, and a vicious cycle can be created. Learning to relax has to be built into a daily pattern based on a healthy diet, regular exercise and a calming routine to wind down before bedtime.

It is important to reduce your intake of stimulating drinks such as tea or coffee, and to avoid eating late at night. It is also helpful to create a relaxing ritual to prepare for falling asleep, with a pleasantly warm evening bath to which you have added your chosen blend of sedative oils. Just experiencing a fragrance that you enjoy will help you to unwind after a long day.

RECOMMENDED ESSENTIAL OILS

Chamomile, clary sage, lavender, marjoram, mandarin, neroli, orange, rose, rosewood and sandalwood.

For sleeplessness following bad dreams:
Blend frankincense, lemon or ylang ylang
with any of the above oils.

Blends for relaxing bath oils:
4 drops rose and 3 drops sandalwood or
5 drops lavender and 3 drops ylang ylang.

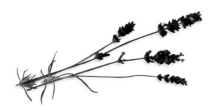

A GENTLE WAVE

The following sequence of strokes washes over the limbs and extremities of the body in outward flowing motions, creating a gentle stream of movement. The soft, downward pulling strokes have a hypnotic and sedative effect, which will calm the emotions and quiet an overactive mind, thereby helping to induce relaxation and sleep.

As you apply the strokes, draw your hands down on the inhalation and pause briefly on the exhalation. This almost imperceptible pause in the motion will create a lovely wave-like feeling, rather than a straight, pulling effect. Each sequence should be performed up to five times on each part of the body.

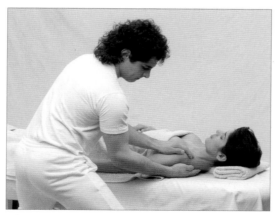

1 Place one hand over the top of the chest, and the other over the muscles on the back of the shoulder, so that the fingers point towards the centre of the body. As you breathe in, pull your hands steadily outwards to the edge of the shoulder and down to just below the joint. Pause briefly as you exhale, letting your hands rest and lightly cradle the top of the arm.

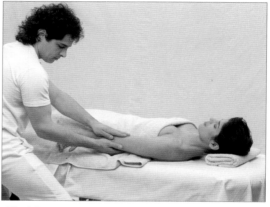

2 Adjust your position so that you can continue the pulling motion down the length of the arm. As you breathe in, pull both hands down to just below the elbow joint. Relax as you breathe out, then continue the slide down the forearm and below the wrist with your next inhalation.

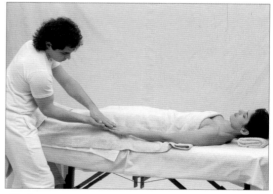

3 Draw your hands over both sides of your partner's hand and fingers, taking your stroke out beyond the body as the hand settles back on to the mattress. Repeat steps 1 to 3 on the other side of the body.

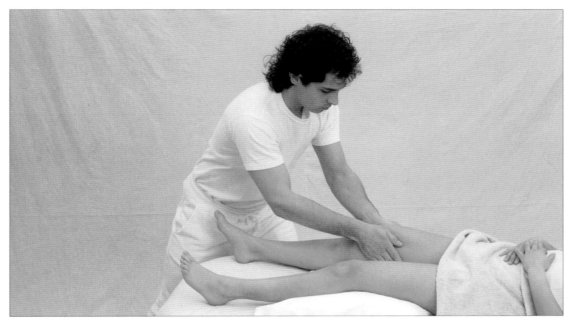

4 Lay both hands slightly above the pelvic girdle to cradle the side of the body. Pull both hands down over the hip socket as you inhale, separating them as they reach the thigh in order to hold each side of the leg; rest briefly as you exhale. With the next inhalation, draw your hands down the leg to just below the knee.

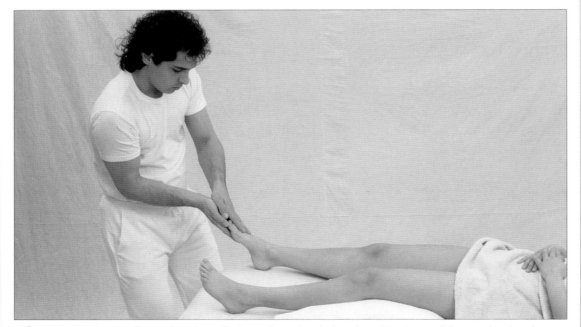

5 Continue this wave-like motion down the lower leg to just below the ankle, then – sliding one hand under the foot with the other on top of the foot – pull gently and steadily out over the toes. Repeat this sequence of strokes on the other side of the body.

SEDATING STROKES ON THE LEGS AND FEET

Finish the sequence with this soothing movement until you feel your partner is relaxed.

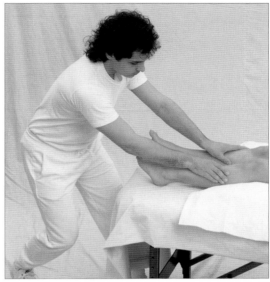

1 Using the flat of both hands, softly stroke down the legs from the thighs until your hands pass over and out of the feet. Repeat the movement as many times as you like to allow your partner to relax.

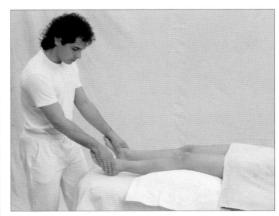

2 To increase the sedative effect of your strokes, complete these sequences with a still, calm hold of your hands over the front of both feet. This will draw the energy down the body, bringing a sense of balance and equilibrium..

ALLEVIATING THE SYMPTOMS OF A COLD

While a cold will normally run its course, combining self-massage with aromatherapy treatment can bring considerable relief from the symptoms. Adding the recommended essential oils to a vaporizer or bowl of steaming water will enable you to inhale their remedial effects, helping to clear the head and soothe the throat and chest, while boosting the immune system.

The foremost treatment for a cold is plenty of rest, which allows the immune system to fight off the viral infection. In the normal course of events a cold usually takes about a week to clear, but if the symptoms persist longer than this, or worsen, it may be advisable to consult your doctor. In the meantime, drink plenty of fluids and increase your intake of fruit and vegetables to help cleanse the body of mucus.

A large number of essential oils can be comforting and helpful in relieving cold symptoms. Tea tree is perhaps the most useful, while eucalyptus is invaluable for relieving a blocked nose and head. All oils are to some extent antiseptic and will assist in preventing the spread of infection. Because most colds present a mixture of symptoms, you should choose one oil for each symptom, then add tea tree to the blend.

INHALING ESSENTIAL OILS

Pour your blended oils into a bowl of hot water and, as they vaporize, inhale the steam as deeply as possible. The oils will begin to decongest blocked nasal passages and soothe the cold symptoms. If you hold a towel over your head this will delay the effects of evaporation. Be careful to place the bowl in a safe position.

RECOMMENDED ESSENTIAL OILS

For the early stages of a cold:
Nutmeg.

For a runny cold:
Ginger.

For bronchitis:
Cedarwood, eucalyptus, frankincense, neroli, orange, peppermint, rosemary, sandalwood.

To loosen catarrh:
Cypress, frankincense, jasmine, lemon, black pepper, sandalwood.

To free congestion:
Frankincense, lemon, eucalyptus.

To boost the immune system:
Bergamot, grapefruit, lavender, lemon, marjoram, rosewood.

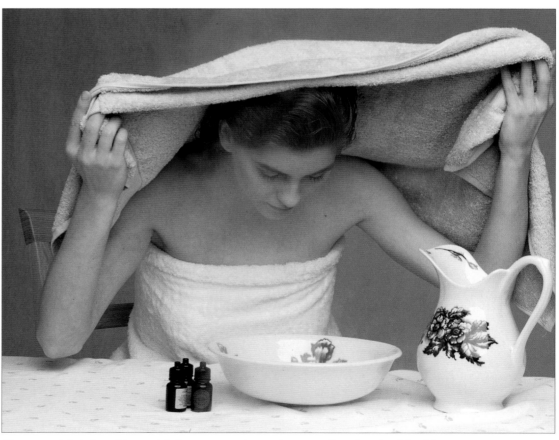

Try a steam inhalation with essential oils to treat nasal congestion or to relieve the pain of sinusitis.

SELF-MASSAGE FOR A COLD

After a steam inhalation, apply some self-massage strokes and pressure on specific points to relieve blocked sinuses.

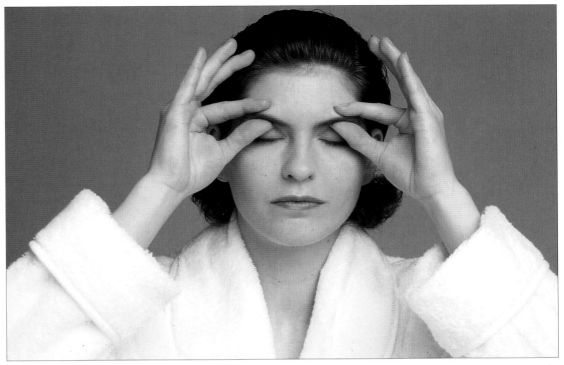

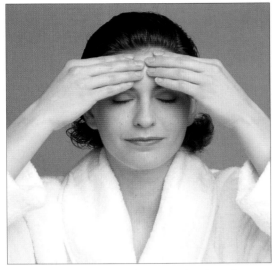

1 Massage all over your brow, starting from the centre and working out with small circular motions from your fingertips.

2 Release pressure from the sinus passages by pinching along the ridge of your eyebrows with your thumbs and index fingers, starting on the inside corners and working, step by step, to the outer edges.

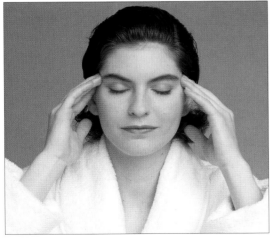

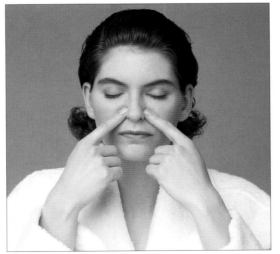

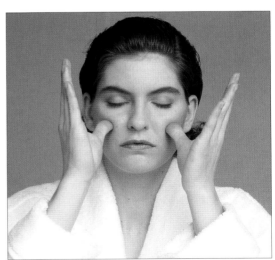

3 Stroke your temples with your fingertips, moving them over the area in circular motions. This will alleviate the stuffiness that can lead to headaches.

4 To relieve congested nasal passages, use your fingertips to press gently into each side of the outer rim of the nostrils at the edge of the cheek-bones. Hold for a count of five and then slowly release the pressure.

5 The small indentations beneath the ridges of the cheekbones indicate the location of some of the sinus passages. Apply thumb pressure slowly up into the hollows. Hold for a count of five and release. This will help clear the head.

MASSAGE THERAPIES TO AID DIGESTION

Emotional tension can cause us to tighten our abdominal muscles and reduce our breathing in order to avoid the experience of painful or uncomfortable feelings. If we are unable to assimilate those emotions, or express them appropriately, they can manifest themselves as physical disorders, particularly playing havoc with the digestive system.

RECOMMENDED ESSENTIAL OILS

To accelerate a sluggish digestion:
Peppermint, black pepper, palmarosa, nutmeg.

For flatulence:
Bergamot, black pepper, fennel, ginger, lemon, marjoram, neroli, nutmeg, peppermint, rosemary.

To soothe colicky pain:
Bergamot, chamomile, clary sage, ginger, cypress, lemon, orange, peppermint, sandalwood.

Constipation:
Black pepper, fennel, ginger, marjoram, neroli, nutmeg, orange, peppermint, rose.

Diarrhoea:
Cypress, chamomile, ginger, lemon, orange, peppermint, black pepper.

A blend for indigestion, colic and flatulence:
1 drop peppermint, 3 drops each of ginger, lemon and bergamot.

Blends for a relaxing compress:
To a bowl of hot water, add 2 drops orange and 3 drops peppermint, or 3 drops chamomile and 2 drops orange.

The key to eliminating indigestion caused by tension is to allow our bodies to let go of such worries and anxieties, and aromatherapy can help a great deal to achieve this. One of the easiest ways to use oils in this context is to disperse them in a bowl of hot water, then make a hot compress and place it over the abdomen, keeping the area warm for up to 10 minutes.

HOLDING AND BREATHING

Still, calm holds over the abdominal area will encourage deeper breathing, allowing the release of pent-up emotions and stress. The following holds will all help to promote relaxation and eliminate tension, enabling the digestive tract to function properly.

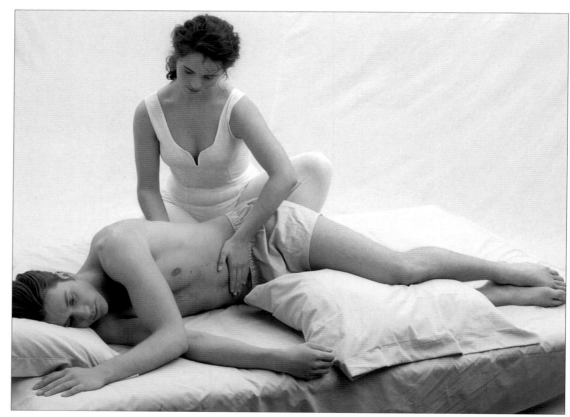

1 If your partner is under extreme stress and is experiencing abdominal pain, ask him to lie on his side with his knees drawn up slightly. Put pillows under his head and between his knees to create a feeling of security. Place one hand over the lower back and the other on his belly, and ask him to breathe slowly and deeply from the abdomen. When the abdominal muscles are relaxed, rub the belly with gentle clockwise strokes.

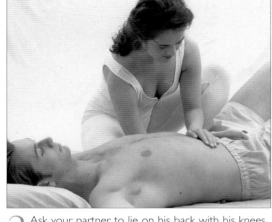

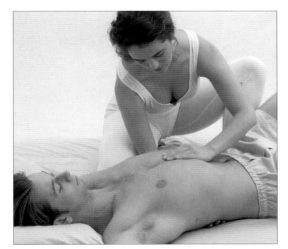

2 Ask your partner to lie on his back with his knees raised. Place one hand under the small of his back and ask him to drop the weight of his pelvis towards your hand. Place your other hand over the abdomen so that its warmth helps to dissolve constriction in the muscles. Then ask your partner to direct his breathing towards your hands and to imagine that each breath is helping the belly to expand and release tension.
Then move your top hand to hold different parts of the abdomen.

3 Encourage deep but gentle breathing in the abdomen and solar plexus region by placing one hand behind the back and the other over the top of the abdomen to encourage the release of tension that can lead to digestive problems. As the area relaxes, gently massage the abdomen with circular strokes of your palm.

RELIEVING ABDOMINAL CRAMP

Passive movements can also be used to reduce the tension which leads to abdominal tightness and pain. You can help to relieve cramp in your partner's belly by pushing his knees towards him. Ask your partner to bend his knees, keeping his feet on the mattress. Adjust your own posture so that you can lean your weight forward as you perform this passive movement. Encourage your partner to give up to you all control of the weight and movement of his legs and concentrate on breathing more deeply. Slowly push the knees towards the trunk of the body, taking care not to force them beyond their natural point of resistance. Help to lower your partner's feet to the mattress, then repeat the movement twice more.

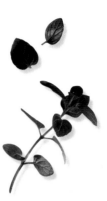

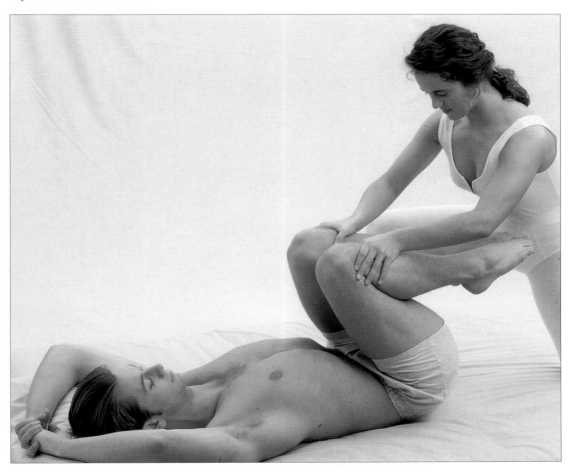

IMPROVING CIRCULATION

A healthy circulatory system is vital to the well-being of both mind and body. Massage with stimulating essential oils, combined with a healthy diet and exercise, is an excellent way of boosting both blood and lymph circulation in order to promote health and vitality.

The circulatory system is divided into two parts: blood circulation, pumped by the heart, and lymph fluid circulation, moved by muscle action. The lymphatic system carries waste products to the lymph nodes, which act as filters to prevent harmful substances from entering the bloodstream, and is an important part of the body's immune defence system.

Poor circulation may be caused by hereditary factors, but it is also affected by a sedentary lifestyle, smoking, an unhealthy diet or emotional stress and tension. A sluggish circulation will cause a depletion of vital nutrients in the body, leading to exhaustion, ill-health, and even depression as toxins build up and the elimination process is impeded. Stimulating essential oils can help to counteract this process and tone up the circulatory system.

RECOMMENDED ESSENTIAL OILS

To stimulate circulation:
Benzoin, black pepper, cedarwood, cypress, eucalyptus, geranium, grapefruit, lemon, mandarin, neroli, rose, rosemary.

To detoxify:
Black pepper, eucalyptus, fennel.

Blend one or more of the stimulant oils with one of the detoxifying oils listed above to treat the problem of poor circulation fully.

BOOSTING AND DRAINING

The signs of a sluggish circulation include pale, mottled or blue-tinged skin, which is usually cold to the touch. The most common areas of poor circulation are the extremities. Lift the limb and apply flowing strokes to boost and drain the blood supply on its return to the heart.

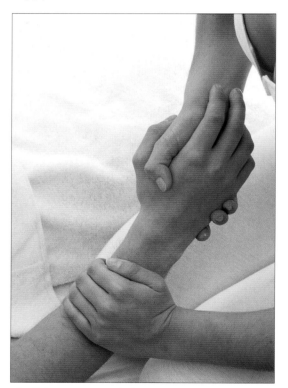

1 Raise your partner's forearm and clasp his hand. Wrap the other hand over the back of the wrist and drain firmly down the arm towards the elbow with a long steady stroke. Glide lightly around the elbow and back up to the wrist. Swap hands to repeat the movement on the inner forearm.

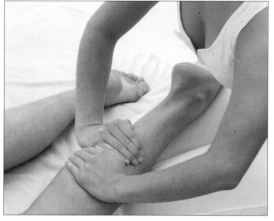

2 Help to increase vitality in the legs and feet by first applying the basic effleurage stroke from the ankle to the back of the knee, with the lower leg in a raised position. Wrap both hands over the back of the ankle, little fingers leading, and firmly stroke up the calf. This position also helps to drain excess water from around puffy ankles.

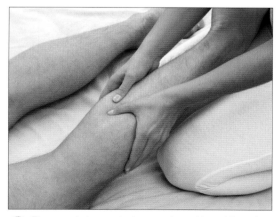

3 Deeper drainage strokes can be achieved by using your thumbs to stroke, in alternating short slides, from the ankle to just below the back of the knee. Repeat several times.

WARMING UP

Hands and feet that are cold as a result of poor circulation can be warmed up by briskly rubbing them between both hands. The friction produces heat and stimulates the blood supply.

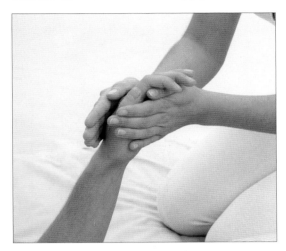

STROKING TOWARDS LYMPH NODES

Gentle, upward effleurage strokes towards the major superficial lymph nodes – such as those in the back of the knee – can assist the lymphatic circulatory system to eliminate toxins from the body, particularly after kneading, friction and deep tissue massage.

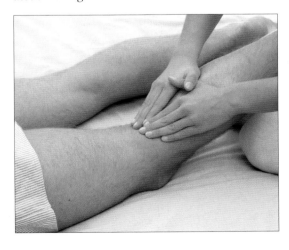

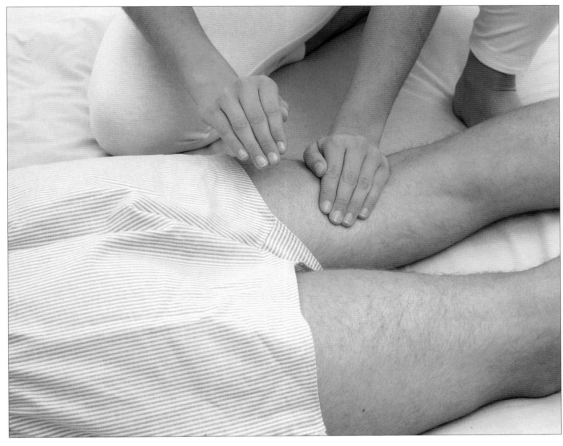

BENEFITING THE SKIN

Pale, flaccid skin benefits from the stimulating effects of all percussion strokes. In particular, the suction effect of cupping draws the blood up towards the skin, bringing vital oxygen and nutrients to its peripheral nerve endings and underlying tissues.

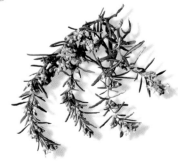

VARICOSE VEINS

The return of de-oxygenated blood to the heart from the lower half of the leg is against the pull of gravity, and some veins have valves in them that open and close to prevent back-flow. When a valve is damaged the veins become dilated causing the condition known as varicose veins. This condition can be exacerbated by pregnancy, obesity, or prolonged standing

It is not advisable to massage directly above or below a varicose vein, but gentle upward-flowing effleurage over the sides of the leg, or away from the damaged vein, will ensure that the area is not neglected during massage. Essential oil blends that improve the circulation will help, but if varicose veins are a result of pregnancy you should not use any oils that are contra-indicated at this time.

DISPERSING CELLULITE AND DETOXIFICATION

Cellulite, which collects mostly on the hips, buttocks and upper arms, is not specifically related to body weight and affects people of all sizes, especially women. It is caused by the accumulation of toxic deposits in the fatty tissues and is detectable by the bumpy "orange peel" look of the skin in these problem areas.

A build-up of cellulite usually results from a sluggish circulation and poor elimination of toxins from the body. To improve the condition it is necessary to use a combination of approaches. Review your diet and cut down on the intake of toxins such as refined carbohydrates, caffeine and alcohol. Increase the amount of fresh vegetables and water. Fennel tea is a natural diuretic which will aid the elimination of toxins. Regular exercise is also important, as it helps the lymphatic system rid the body of waste products.

Massage with the recommended essential oils should become part of your daily routine for 6–8 weeks to help achieve a smooth and healthy skin. Mechanical massage instruments are helpful for this. You can try a quick self-massage several times a day, such as when dressing or after taking a bath or shower. Squeeze and knead the thighs and buttocks, and follow up with a range of percussion movements to shift fatty deposits under the skin.

RECOMMENDED ESSENTIAL OILS

To stimulate and detoxify:
Black pepper, eucalyptus, fennel.

To stimulate circulation and prevent water retention:
Geranium, lemon, grapefruit.

Blend 3 drops lemon, 2 drops geranium, 2 drops fennel and 1 drop black pepper in 10 ml/2 tsp carrier oil.

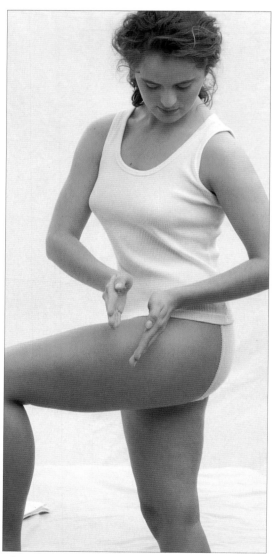

SELF-MASSAGE

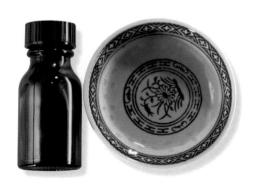

1 Hand-held massage instruments such as this wooden six-ball roller are ideal for making the circular pressure motions that help to smooth out cellulite spots on the thighs.

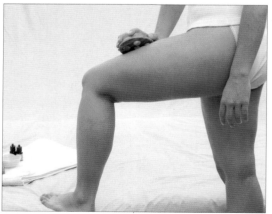

2 Hack, cup and pummel the thighs briskly to tone the area and revitalize the blood circulation.

CELLULITE REDUCTION MASSAGE

If cellulite is a problem, focus your attention on the problem areas of the thighs and buttocks when giving a massage to boost the blood supply to the tissues and help to increase the lymphatic drainage of waste products.

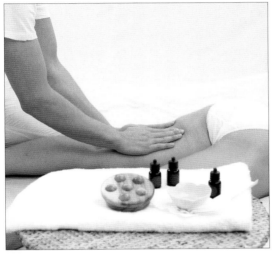

1 Soothe, warm and relax the thigh muscles with upward flowing effleurage strokes such as integration and fanning motions. Repeat several times, always returning the stroke to the back of the knee by gliding your hands around and down the sides of the leg.

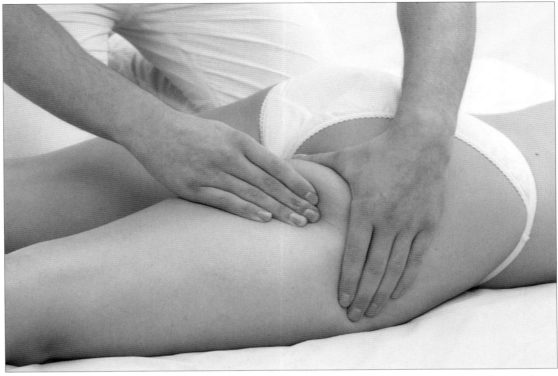

2 Knead thoroughly over the whole area to enliven the thigh and buttock muscles and help the exchange of tissue fluids. Follow up with effleurage strokes to boost the circulation.

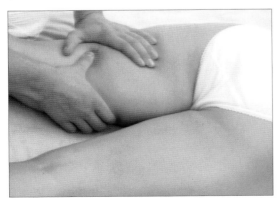

3 Deep friction strokes help to break up toxic deposits. Squeeze and rotate your thumb on one area at a time, using your other hand to push the tissue towards the stroke. Follow these strokes with fanning motions to aid the elimination process.

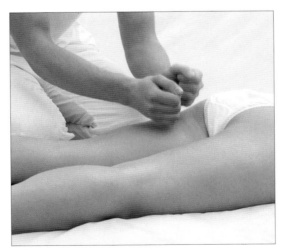

4 Pummel, hack and cup the thigh and buttocks, one hand following the other in rapid succession, flicking off the skin at the moment of contact.

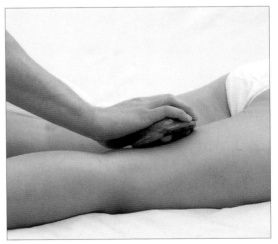

5 Soothe the thighs and buttocks with effleurage strokes. If you have a mechanical roller, use it to add to the benefits of your cellulite massage by moving it in circular motions. This is particularly effective when the skin is oiled.

AROMATHERAPY IN PREGNANCY

Pregnancy can be one of the most exciting and fulfilling times of a woman's life. The joy of bringing another human being into the world creates a tremendous feeling of contentment and anticipation, but it is also a time of great physical and emotional upheaval. Together with the ever-important trio of exercise, good diet and rest, essential oils can play an important role in helping a woman cope with the stresses of pregnancy, the pain of labour and post-natal recovery.

RECOMMENDED ESSENTIAL OILS

Chamomile, geranium (in low doses), lavender, lemon, neroli, orange, rose, sandalwood.

For nausea:
Black pepper, ginger, lemon, nutmeg, rosewood, sandalwood.

To counteract heartburn:
Peppermint, lemon.

To combat fluid retention:
Geranium, grapefruit, mandarin, neroli, orange.

To tone the system in preparation for labour:
Geranium.

For lower back massage during labour:
Geranium, lemon, neroli.

For lower back massage in late pregnancy, lend 4 drops each lavender and sandalwood in 30 ml/2 tbsp carrier oil.

Spoil yourself with the luxurious and relaxing scent of rose for body and facial oils to keep your spirits up during pregnancy.

BLENDS AND REMEDIES FOR COMMON AILMENTS

Aromatherapy can help with many of the minor problems that may occur during pregnancy.

Heartburn

Avoid heavy meals and rich, spicy foods. Peppermint tea infusions help, or rub the solar plexus with a blend of 2 drops each lemon and peppermint in 15 ml/1 tbsp carrier oil.

Constipation

Make sure you eat plenty of fresh, high-fibre foods and drink plenty of still water. Tension can be a contributory factor, so try a relaxing bath with 3 drops lavender and 4 drops rose oil. Massage the abdomen and back with 4 drops chamomile or orange in 15 ml/1 tbsp carrier oil.

Sleep problems

A relaxing bath with 3 drops each neroli and rose will help you to get a good night's sleep, and you can add 2 drops ylang ylang for its calming, sedative effect. A couple of drops of rose or lavender on the pillow will help.

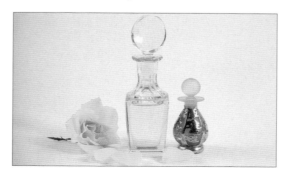

Sore breasts

These need extra care during pregnancy as they expand. Use gentle massage with 3 drops each rose and orange in 15 ml/1 tsbp sweet almond oil, or make a cool rose-water compress if your breasts are swollen. Sweet almond oil on its own is excellent for sore or cracked nipples during breast-feeding. Never use pure essential oils on the breasts during this period as they can easily be transferred to the baby during feeding.

Stretch marks

A daily massage around the hips and expanding tummy, using 2 drops mandarin and 1 drop neroli, or 5 drops lavender in 15 ml/1 tbsp jojoba, wheat germ or evening primrose oil, will help keep skin supple. Start around the fifth month and continue after the birth until you return to your normal weight.

Swollen ankles

Weight gain and fluid retention may result in swollen ankles. These can be reduced with a lukewarm footbath containing 2 drops each benzoin, rose and orange. Rest with feet raised whenever possible.

Varicose veins

Mix 2 drops each cypress, lemongrass and lavender into 30 ml/2 tbsp apricot kernel oil and smooth gently over the legs to give relief. If the veins are prominent, one of the best oils for the circulation is geranium, but this should always be very dilute for use during pregnancy. Add a maximum of 4 drops to the bath or to 15 ml/1 tbsp carrier oil to massage the leg with upward movements. Do not work directly over the veins or apply too much pressure.

EASING LOWER BACK STRAIN

Pregnancy can put a great deal of strain on the curvature of the lower spine and the surrounding muscles, sometimes leading to chronic back pain. Focus massage strokes on the lower back and buttocks, enabling the area to release its tension.

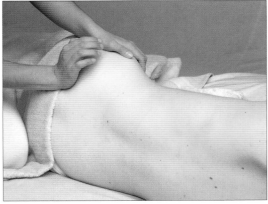

1 Spread oil over the lower back and buttocks, warming and soothing the muscles with soft effleurage strokes. Then begin to work deeper into the gluteal muscles of the buttocks, rotating the heel of the hand in one area at a time while supporting the hip with the other hand.

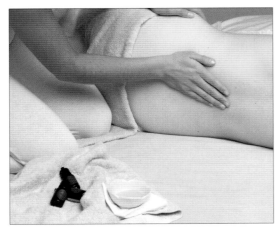

2 A pregnant woman will instinctively place a hand over the base of her spine to soothe away pain. Bring relief to the muscles surrounding and covering the pelvic girdle and lower back with flowing, circular motions from the surface of your hand.

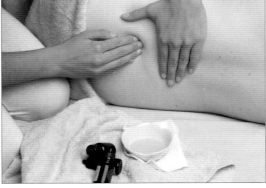

3 Tiny, circular friction movements with the finger-tips will deepen the remedial effects of strokes on the lower back. Ease away tension in the muscle that covers the sacrum, the flat triangular bone at the base of the spine, pushing the tissue towards the stroke with the other hand.

CIRCLING THE ABDOMEN

After the first three months of a healthy pregnancy, the abdomen can be gently massaged with soft circular movements. The warmth of your touch and the soporific motions will be very relaxing to both the mother and the baby.

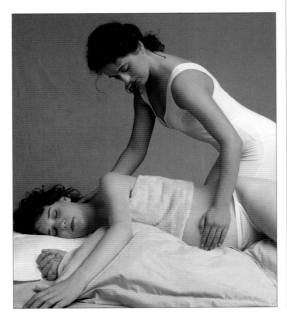

LABOUR

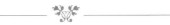

To create a relaxing atmosphere, use a few drops of lavender in a vaporizer or try rose, neroli or ylang ylang to fortify you as time passes. If labour is progressing slowly, try marjoram in a massage oil or compress to stimulate contractions.

AFTER THE BIRTH

The "baby blues" often occur around the third or fourth day after birth, though some women can suffer a more severe form of post-natal depression for much longer. A bath with jasmine and ylang ylang will help you to feel better, or add a blend of chamomile, geranium and orange to a body oil to help with hormonal imbalance.

A bath with lavender will soothe perineal soreness. Add tea tree for its antiseptic properties.

CAUTIONS: The following oils should be avoided during pregnancy (particularly during the first five months) because of their strong diuretic properties, or tendency to induce menstruation: *bay, basil, clary sage, comfrey, fennel, hyssop, juniper, marjoram, melissa, myrrh, rosemary, thyme, sage.*

Use all essential oils in half the usual quantity during pregnancy and take extra care in handling them. Ensure that the oils you are using are pure essential oils, as adulterated blends or synthetic oils can sometimes have less predictable effects.

If you have a history of miscarriage you should also avoid chamomile and lavender for the first few months, although in general they are excellent oils for pregnancy.

Because of their potentially toxic nature and strong abortive qualities, the following oils should never be used except by a qualified aromatherapist, and must be avoided during pregnancy: *oreganum, pennyroyal, St John's wort, tansy, wormwood.*

BABY MASSAGE

*All babies thrive on being cuddled, touched and massaged, for skin-to-skin contact is essential to the nurturing of a baby,
helping her to bond with her parents and to develop emotional and physical health and self-esteem. Massage and touch
can become a natural part of play with a young baby, especially during and after bath time, or before she is dressed.
No formal routine is needed, just gently stroke the baby's body and limbs, using effleurage circles and fanning motions.
Alternatively, softly squeeze, knead and perform passive movements on the arms, legs, fingers and toes. Your touch will
comfort and soothe the baby, helping her to explore and discover the wonders of her body.*

RECOMMENDED ESSENTIAL OILS

It is both safe and beneficial to use essential oils with babies and young children, as long as you ensure that the dosage is correctly prepared and you exercise common sense when selecting the oils. As a precaution, avoid the very stimulating, strong-smelling oils.

For newborn babies
For fretfulness:
Chamomile, geranium, lavender, mandarin.

For nappy rash and skin irritation:
Chamomile, lavender.

For cradle cap:
Eucalyptus (Eucalyptus radiata), geranium.

For teething:
Chamomile, lavender.
Dosage: 1–3 drops of essential oil in
30 ml/2 tbsp carrier oil.

For babies from 2–6 months
All the above oils are effective for babies
of this age, as well as mandarin and neroli.
For sickness, peppermint may be calming:
put 1 drop on a cotton wool ball at the foot
of the baby's cot.

CAUTION: Do not use peppermint for babies
under 2 months. In cases of sickness you could
try spearmint as an alternative.
Dosage: 3–5 drops of essential oil in
30 ml/2 tbsp carrier oil.

For babies from 6–12 months
In addition to the oils suggested above,
grapefruit, palmarosa and tea tree can be used.
For hyperactive children, essential oil of
marjoram can be very helpful, but as this
problem is usually complex it is important
that you should seek the advice of
your doctor as well.
Dosage: 3–5 drops of essential oil in
30 ml/2 tbsp carrier oil.

To alleviate the symptoms of coughs
and colds in babies and children
of all ages:
*Eucalyptus, lavender and tea tree in
a vaporizer.*

SOOTHING AND FEATHERING

This routine will help the parent and baby form a loving, secure relationship.

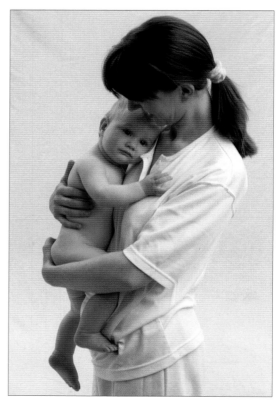

1 Hold your baby close to you so she can feel the
warmth of your body, the beat of your heart and
the rhythm of your breathing, enabling her to melt into
you and be comforted by your familiar presence.

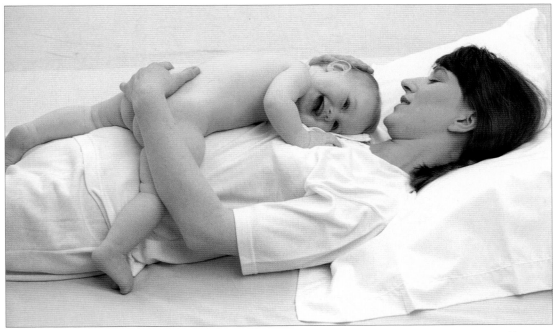

2 Babies love to lie against the softness of your body. Soothe her by placing one hand over the base of her spine, while gently stroking her head.

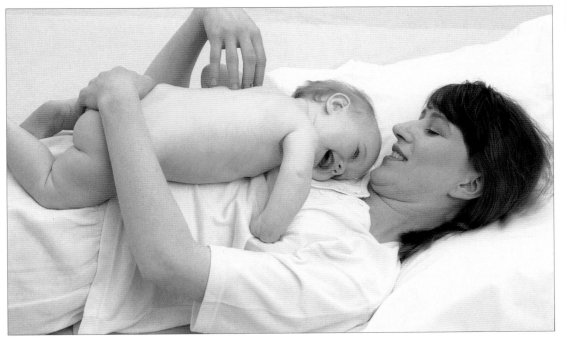

3 Running your fingertips up and down the baby's back will make her giggle with pleasure as the featherlike touches brush her delicate skin.

EFFLEURAGE

If the baby can keep still for long enough, you can rub nourishing oil into her skin while giving her a massage. Soft effleurage strokes on her back, such as fanning and circles, will delight her.

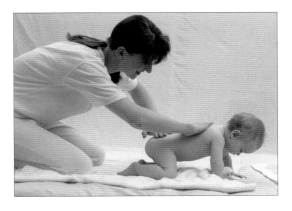

KNEADING AND SQUEEZING

Chubby little arms and legs are made for gentle kneading and squeezing. Press the limbs softly between your thumb and fingers.

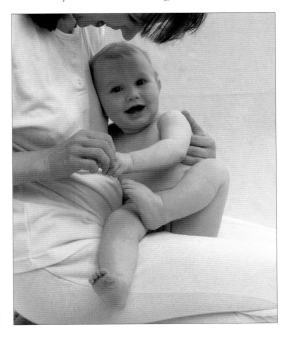

MASSAGE FOR THE ELDERLY

Many elderly people live full and active lives, and aromatherapy massage provides a valuable contribution to the maintenance of their physical and emotional health. The contact of touch through the medium of massage is especially important for alleviating feelings of isolation, which may result from loneliness or bereavement.

Using essential oils for the elderly presents no particular difficulties, but it is advisable to bear in mind two general points. First, as we age our metabolism slows down, so that any chemical introduced into the body will remain there slightly longer. Second, because of this slower metabolic rate and a less physically active life, the whole system can become more toxic. This is particularly true for those people who must necessarily live a more sedentary life through disability, or are in residential homes or hospitals.

It is best to avoid the highly stimulating oils and make use of those with gentler effects. A more dilute blend may also be advisable.

Whole body massage is beneficial to older people, but if they are uncomfortable about undressing, then massage on the hands, feet and face can also be helpful. Still, hands-on holds, to induce feelings of calm and peace, can be applied to the body just as well while the person is fully clothed.

Regular hand and footbaths with essential oils are an excellent preventive measure against stiff and aching joints in the extremities.

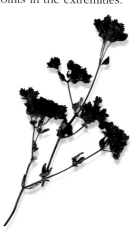

STILL HANDS-ON HOLDS

A condition commonly affecting the elderly is the onset of osteoarthritis, a degenerative disease of the joints caused by wear and tear. One or several joints of the body may be affected. Gentle massage with the recommended essential oils brings great relief. However, it is not advisable to massage over the joints if they are inflamed, swollen or disintegrated. In these circumstances, still holds will allow the warmth of your hands to subtly comfort the affected area, helping to increase circulation and reduce stiffness.

RECOMMENDED ESSENTIAL OILS

Frankincense, geranium, ginger, grapefruit, jasmine, juniper, lavender, marjoram, nutmeg, neroli, rosemary, sandalwood.

For arthritis:
Benzoin, black pepper, chamomile, cedarwood, eucalyptus, ginger, juniper, lemon, marjoram, nutmeg.

For aches and pains:
Ginger.

For grief and loneliness:
Marjoram, rose, nutmeg.

For constipation:
Black pepper, fennel, ginger, marjoram.

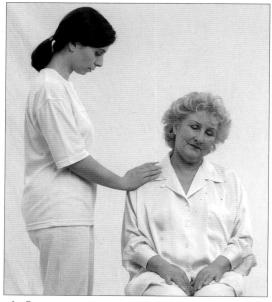

1 Focus your attention and breath into your hands before gently cradling the shoulder. This supportive hold will help the shoulder relax.

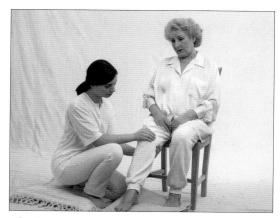

2 Osteoarthritis commonly affects the knee joints in older people. Cup the knee between your hands to bring it warmth and comfort.

RELAXING THE SPINE

Long periods of sitting still may cause tension and stiffness in the spine.

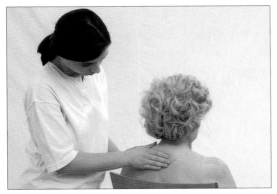

1 Soft, circular effleurage strokes over the top of the spine, at the base of the neck and between the shoulder blades, will ease away tension. While massaging with one hand, use the other hand to support the front of the body.

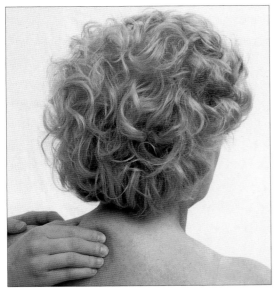

2 Excess tissue frequently builds up over stiff, tense areas, further inhibiting flexibility. Once the muscles are warmed with effleurage, sink into a deeper level of tissue with friction strokes. Use small circular motions from your fingertips to loosen and stretch the areas surrounding the top of the spine.

STAYING SUPPLE

Massaging the hands and feet will help to keep the wrists, fingers, ankles and toes supple, giving the whole system an extra boost.

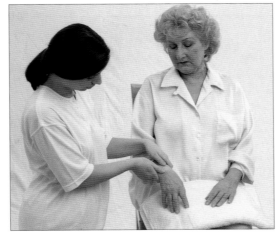

1 Support the wrist with your fingers, and apply circular and sliding strokes with your thumbs to ease away tension from its tiny bones.

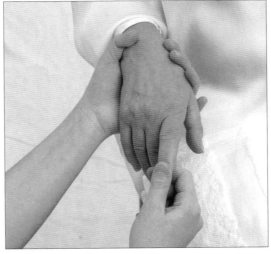

2 Many older people wish to pursue their hobbies, which may require dextrous hands and fingers. If the joints are not inflamed or degenerated, regular hand massage, with gentle passive movements and stretching of the fingers, will assist this continued flexibility in the hands.

A SOOTHING NECK AND FACE MASSAGE

This is an excellent way of easing away physical and emotional tension in elderly people. The loving contact of your hands is especially comforting in times of loneliness, distress or bereavement.

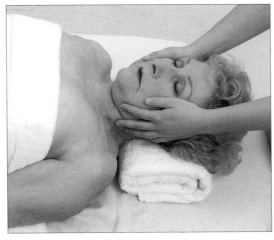

Support the head with a cushion or folded towel and apply gentle circular and sliding strokes with your fingertips to the neck and face working upwards to the hairline.

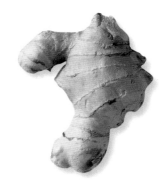

CONVALESCENCE AND RECUPERATION

*After an illness or injury the body is left in a vulnerable condition, and a period of convalescence is vital to give the
immune system time to rebuild its defences. Massage helps to promote this important transition from a period when
the body is battling to heal itself to full recovery and a return to normal health.*

The period of convalescence is usually a time of physical and emotional fluctuation. The patient may experience bursts of energy, followed by fatigue when the spirits fall. Gentle, hands-on holds are ideal for the first fragile stages of convalescence. The touch of your hands will comfort the body, stimulating the nerves that replenish the vital organs, and return the body to a normal resting state. As your partner recuperates, whole body massage will tone up the muscles, boosting circulation and increasing the body's overall vitality and sense of well-being.

RECOMMENDED ESSENTIAL OILS

To stimulate the appetite:
Black pepper, orange.

To overcome lethargy:
Black pepper, tea tree.

To comfort and lift the spirits:
Orange, nutmeg.

To boost the immune system:
Bergamot, black pepper, rosewood, tea tree.

Tonics: *Clary sage, mandarin.*

HEALING HOLDS

These soothing holds help to balance the nervous system and increase the body's energy levels. Your caring touch will stimulate the skin senses and help to restore emotional health and self-esteem, vital to the healing process. Start at the head, gently placing your hands over the forehead, temples and cheeks, then work methodically down both sides of the body to the feet. Proceed in a relaxed and unhurried manner, giving equal attention to all parts of the body.

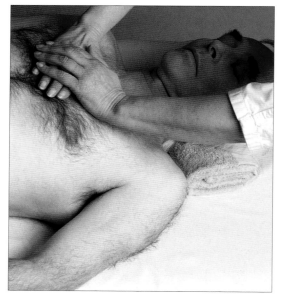

2 Slowly withdraw your left hand and rest it on top of your right hand. Tune in to the heartbeat and the rise and fall of the breath.

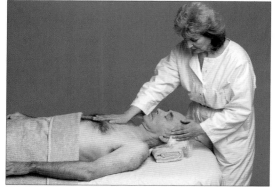

1 Gently cup your left hand over your partner's temple and place your right hand over the heart area. This helps to encourage a sense of integration between mind and body.

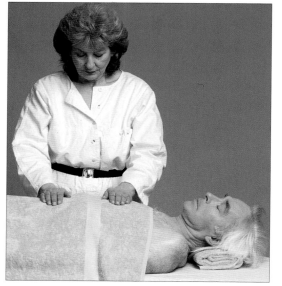

3 Move to the side and rest one hand on the chest and one over the solar plexus. This helps to decrease anxiety and encourages deeper breathing.

CLEARING THE HEAD

A prolonged period of inactivity can cause the shoulder and neck muscles to tense up, restricting the circulation which, in turn, leads to headaches. Relax the shoulder and neck area by kneading the shoulders, then follow this with a neck, head and face massage.

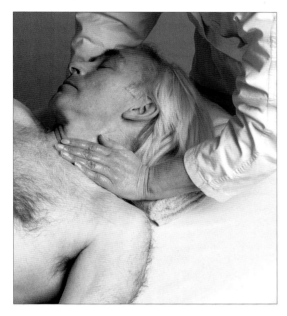

GETTING READY FOR ACTION

As your partner recuperates and becomes stronger, he will be eager to resume normal activities. When he has reached this stage in his convalescence, focus your massage on the feet and legs to boost a sluggish circulatory system, and massage the arms and hands to renew their strength and dexterity.

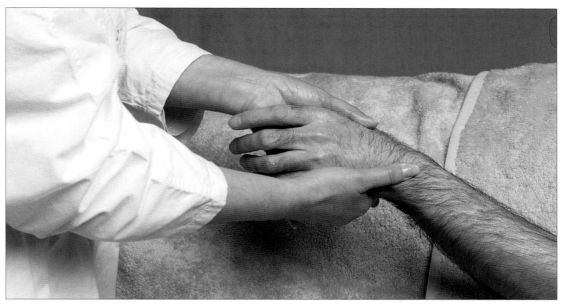

1 Massage the hands and fingers to release tension and increase flexibility. Use circular and sliding strokes with your thumbs and stretch the fingers gently.

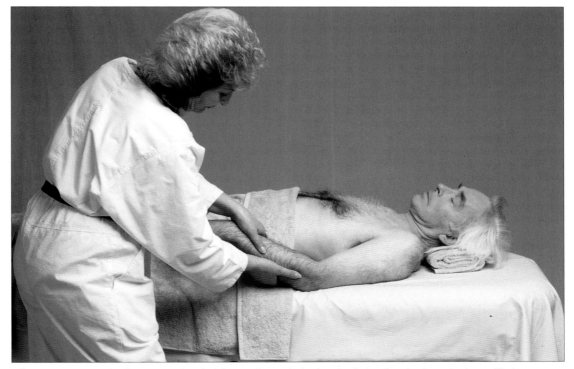

2 Now massage the forearms, using draining strokes to help the circulation flow back to the heart. To loosen and warm the muscles, use one hand after the other in a fanning motion, working towards the elbow.

DEVELOPING YOUR KNOWLEDGE

*Once you have become familiar with essential oils and with the practical benefits they offer, you may wish to gain
a deeper understanding of the nature of these aromatic substances.*

Most people begin to collect essential oils slowly, one by one, as they can afford them. You will usually choose oils to answer a particular need, or because you find a scent especially appealing. Having used the oils for a while you may become aware that your understanding of the use and benefits of a particular oil has deepened. This may become apparent with the realization that the aroma of the oil will relieve a painful or disquieting emotion or a physical symptom time after time. If you would like to explore this situation further, here are two exercises that may help.

ESSENTIAL OILS AND YOUR STATE OF MIND

The power essential oils possess to affect our state of mind is available to all of us if we actively choose to use them for one of these specific purposes. A suitable occasion might be prior to a very special social event, an interview or exam, or a period of study. You may also want to refresh yourself after an unpleasant experience such as an argument or an unwelcome visitor. The relaxing oils are helpful when preparing for meditation, or to clear the mind before going to sleep.

EXERCISE ONE

The first exercise uses the power of the imagination to take you on a journey inspired by an oil of your choice. You will need to choose a period of at least half an hour when you will not be interrupted. Find a comfortable upright chair, or a cushion on which you can sit comfortably on the floor; the essential oil of your choice, preferably one that you have used frequently for a reasonable period of time; and a handkerchief or paper tissue.

Put 1–2 drops of your chosen essential oil on to the handkerchief or tissue and place it within easy reach. Seat yourself comfortably. If you are sitting in a chair you may want to put a cushion under your feet to help you relax. Once you are in a comfortable position place your hands lightly, palms down, on your thighs. Concentrate on the rise and fall of your breath and become observant of your breath as it enters and leaves your body. If any thoughts of daily activities come into your head, acknowledge them and then allow them to pass away.

After a few minutes have passed, take the scented handkerchief and inhale from it deeply for one or two breaths. Try to observe which parts of the body you become aware of and what feelings are there – for example, it may be a warm sensation or a tingling one. Colours may come to mind, specific pictures, or perhaps a dream-like story. Allow the inspiration of the scent to transport you in your imagination, and as far as possible allow yourself really to trust what you imagine and feel. When the images begin to fade, gently bring your attention back to your own breathing, observing the rise and fall of your chest.

Become aware again of the comfortable chair in the room and, when you are completely ready, slowly open your eyes. You may feel a little dreamy after completing the exercise, and a glass

The stress that is often associated with periods of unusually hard work, or studying for an exam, may be eased by using an essential oil such as ginger or cedarwood.

of water or juice can help regain a solid, present feeling in your body. The activity of writing down any thoughts and feelings about the experience will also help achieve this.

By making this journey into the imagination several times with different essential oils it is possible to develop your confidence and intuitive knowledge. As a guide, the whole process should last approximately 15 minutes.

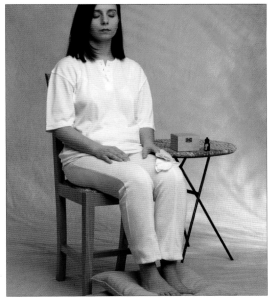

1 Choose a time when you will not be disturbed. Make sure you adopt a comfortable position, and put everyday concerns out of your mind.

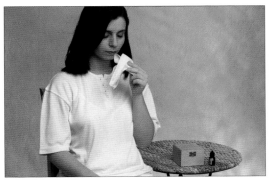

2 When your mind is clear, take the handkerchief or tissue with the essential oil on it and inhale for one or two breaths.

EXERCISE TWO

The second exercise provides an alternative way of getting to know each essential oil in greater depth. You will need to have the bathroom to yourself for half an hour or more. You will also need the essential oil or oils of your choice, a candle securely fixed in a holder and some matches. Some people like to listen to a relaxing piece of music while bathing, so you may like to have this ready too.

Try to do this exercise at a time when you don't need to cleanse yourself thoroughly, so that the bath is purely relaxing. Run as deep a bath as you can, making sure the water is at a comfortable temperature. Meanwhile, blend the essential oils in a carrier oil.

When you are ready, concentrate on the purpose of the bath and light the candle. Put the blended essential oil into the bath just before you get into it. Remain in the bath for as long as you feel like it, or until the water is no longer comfortably warm. Allow any thoughts that float into your mind to come and go gently, and concentrate on any dreamlike images or colours inspired by the aromas rising in the steam.

This type of bath can be tremendously restorative as well as developing a heightened awareness of each of the oils you use in this way.

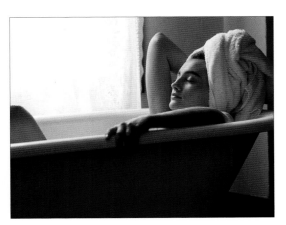

Enjoy your aromatherapy bath as a relaxation exercise rather than a cleansing routine, with plenty of time to absorb the aromas.

RECOMMENDED ESSENTIAL OILS

For a special occasion:
Clary sage, grapefruit, orange.

In preparation for an exam or interview:
Bergamot, black pepper, cedarwood, frankincense, ginger, grapefruit, lemon, neroli, orange, peppermint, rosemary, rosewood, sandalwood.

To help when studying:
Bergamot, eucalyptus, frankincense, ginger, grapefruit, jasmine, juniper, lemon, peppermint, rosemary, nutmeg.

For cleansing after difficult situations:
Cypress, eucalyptus, juniper, lavender, lemon, peppermint, rosemary.

To aid meditation:
Cedarwood, clary sage, frankincense, jasmine, palmarosa, rosewood, sandalwood.

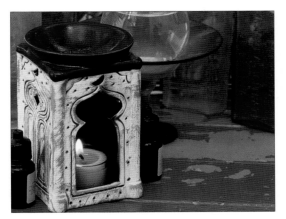

Lighted candles or an aromatherapy burner, with the same oil as you have in the bath, will heighten the atmosphere.

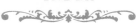
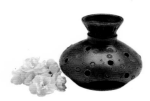

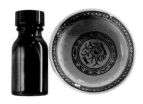